Nutrition and Exercise

CURRENT CONCEPTS IN NUTRITION

Myron Winick, Editor

Institute of Human Nutrition
Columbia University College of Physicians and Surgeons

NUTRITION AND EXERCISE

Edited by

MYRON WINICK

Institute of Human Nutrition
College of Physicians and Surgeons
Columbia University
New York, New York

A WILEY-INTERSCIENCE PUBLICATION

JOHN WILEY & SONS

New York • Chichester • Brisbane • Toronto • Singapore

Library of Congress Cataloging in Publication Data:

Nutrition and exercise.

(Current concepts in nutrition ; v. 15)
"A Wiley-Interscience publication."
Includes index.
1. Exercise—Physiological aspects. 2. Nutrition.
3. Diet therapy. 4. Exercise therapy. I. Winick, Myron. II. Series.
QP301.N87 1986 613.7'1 86-7823
ISBN 0-471-84562-0

Printed in the United States of America

10 9 8 7 6 5 4 3 2 1

Preface

Exercise and nutrition interact at many levels in the maintenance of health and the prevention of disease. This volume discusses this interaction from the standpoint of the biochemical and physiologic changes induced by exercise, the ways in which exercise affects specific populations, and the role of exercise and nutrition in the prevention and treatment of disease. Each chapter is written by an expert in the field, making available the latest research data. At the same time the volume as a whole covers in an integrated manner the entire spectrum of nutrition–exercise interrelations.

The first few chapters focus on the changes induced in the body by exercise and how these changes may alter nutritional requirements. Based on these physiologic considerations a rational approach to exercise prescription is put forth. In Chapter 4, Dr. John Garrow discusses diet and thermogenesis, a topic that has become very important in our understanding of obesity.

The remaining chapters focus on specific populations and disease states, covering women, adolescents, athletes, and such diseases as obesity, atherosclerosis, and diabetes.

This volume is a complete examination of the interaction of exercise and nutrition at a fundamental and clinical level. It is designed for professionals in the field of nutrition, medicine, and exercise physiology as well as those interested in health maintenance and disease prevention.

MYRON WINICK

New York, New York
May 1986

Contents

Nutrition and Exercise

1

Acute and Chronic Metabolism Changes Following Exercise: Mechanisms and Physiological Relevance

N. B. RUDERMAN, M.D., Dphil.,
T. BALON, Ph.D., A. ZORZANO, Ph.D.,
M. N. GOODMAN, Ph.D., and J. YOUNG, Ph.D.

Boston University, Boston, Massachusetts

Vigorous exercise produces the most extreme cardiopulmonary and metabolic perturbations experienced by normal people. Therefore it is not surprising that since the era of Claude Bernard, there has been a great interest in exploring the basis for these perturbations and how they allow us to exercise more effectively. Only more recently, however, has it been appreciated that exercise also produces physiological and metabolic alterations that persist long after physical activity has ceased. In this chapter, we describe some of these alterations as they occur in people who perform endurance exercise on a regular basis. We also present data suggesting that persistent metabolic and hormonal effects can be produced by a single bout of exercise and

Supported in part by USPHS grants AM19514 and TAM00652 and a grant to Dr., Young from Ross Laboratories. The authors thank Eva Belur, Judith Treadway, and Pilar Rivera for their technical assistance and Gretchen Fox for typing the manuscript.

that these, rather than improved fitness, may account for many of the changes seen in trained individuals.

ALTERATIONS WITH ENDURANCE EXERCISE

Perhaps the best known effect of chronic endurance exercise is an increase in one's maximum capacity for aerobic work (VO_2). As reviewed by Holloszy and Booth (1) this is partially due to an increase in the capacity of skeletal muscle to carry out oxidative metabolism. Thus in trained animals and humans, increases in mitochondrial number and size, increased activity of key enzymes of fat and carbohydrate metabolism and the citric acid cycle, and increases in myoglobin and muscle capillarization have all been described. Alterations in the cardiovascular system such as an increase in maximum cardiac output also contribute to the increase in VO_{2max}.

Recently it has been demonstrated that there are also a number of distinctive metabolic and hormonal alterations in endurance athletes. A partial list presented in Table 1-1 includes changes in plasma lipids, increased insulin sensitivity, diminished adiposity, and in some individuals improved glucose tolerance. It is in great measure because of these changes that there has been an intense effort to assess the value of exercise in treating or preventing such disorders as coronary heart disease, diabetes, and obesity.

Table 1-1. A Partial List of Metabolic and Hormonal Adaptations to Endurance Exercise

↓ Triglycerides
↑ HDL cholesterol
↓ LDL cholesterol[a]
↑ Glucose tolerance[a]
↑ Insulin sensitivity
↓ Adiposity

[a]Not always seen. When it occurs may be associated with diminished adiposity.

METABOLIC ALTERATIONS FOLLOWING A SINGLE BOUT OF EXERCISE

Maehlum, Felig, and Wahren (2) demonstrated that after a single bout of exercise, exogenous glucose is taken up predominantly by muscle to replete its glycogen stores, rather than by liver as in the resting state. The basis for this shift in glucose distribution was not examined; however, the fact that it could occur in the absence of a large increase in plasma insulin suggested that the sensitivity of muscle to insulin may have increased.

To test this hypothesis we examined glucose metabolism in previously exercised rats by using a perfused muscle preparation, the isolated rat hindquarter. In initial studies rats fed ad libitum were run on a treadmill for 45 minutes at a rate of 18m/minute (moderate intensity), and approximately 30 minutes after the cessation of exercise their hindquarters were perfused (3). As shown in Table 1-2, when insulin was not added to the perfusing media, glucose uptake was the same in control and previously exercised rats. On the other hand, at insulin concentrations as low as 30 μU/ml glucose utilization was significantly greater in the exercised group. Maximum differences between the groups

Table 1-2. Glucose Utilization by the Isolated Perfused Rat Hindquarter Following Exercise of Moderate Intensity[a]

	Glucose Uptake (μmol/g/h)	
Insulin	No Exercise	Exercise
0	1.8 ± 0.2	1.9 ± 0.4
30	1.9 ± 0.2	2.7 ± 0.2[b]
75	3.2 ± 0.2	6.1 ± 0.3[b]
500	6.3 ± 0.1	9.4 ± 1.1[b]
20,000	10.2 ± 0.9	12.6 ± 0.5[b]

[a]Results are means ± SE of at least three experiments and were obtained during a 45 minute perfusion initiated approximately 30 minutes after the cessation of exercise. Adapted from Richter and coworkers (3).
[b]$p < .05$ when compared to no exercise group.

occurred at an insulin concentration of 75 μU/ml. This increase in insulin effect persisted for at least 4 hours, but was no longer evident at 24 hours. Not shown is that nearly all of the additional glucose taken up by the muscle was used for glycogen synthesis. Also the increase in glycogen synthesis was predominantly restricted to muscles that had been partially depleted of glycogen during the exercise, suggesting regulation by local factors.

Similar studies were performed after more intense exercise (36m/minute for 50 minutes). Exercise in these rats consisted of five runs of 10 minutes each interspersed with 3 minute rest periods. Under these conditions, muscles were more depleted of glycogen at the time they were perfused and glucose utilization by the hindquarter was observed in the absence as well as in the presence of insulin (4). Interestingly when these rats were studied several hours after the cessation of exercise, their muscle glycogen stores were substantially repleted, and only the increase in insulin-stimulated glucose utilization was observed.

From these studies we have concluded that the repletion of muscle glycogen after exercise occurs in two phases: phase I, during which glycogen stores are still depleted and glucose utilization is increased in the absence as well as in the presence of insulin; and phase II, which occurs when glycogen stores are substantially repleted and is associated only with the increase in insulin-stimulated glucose utilization. Presumably phase I corresponds to the period of rapid glycogen repletion immediately after exercise and phase II to the period of supercompensation (4).

The physiological relevance of these phenomena is suggested by recent studies in patients with type II diabetes reported by Schneider and his coworkers (5) in which improved HbA_1 levels during physical training were attributed to the cumulative effect of the individual exercise bouts. Likewise, Heath and coworkers (6) have observed that 10 days of detraining diminishes glucose tolerance and increases the insulin response to a glucose load in highly trained individuals even though their level of fitness (as judged by VO_{2max}) was unchanged. Of particular note in the latter study was the observation that a single bout of exercise after 11 days of detraining restored both glucose tolerance and plasma insulin to their predetraining values on the following day.

INSULIN AND THERMOGENESIS

An increase in thermogenesis has been observed during euglycemic insulin clamp studies in man (7,8) and there have been reports of increased O_2 consumption as long as 24 hours after vigorous exercise (9). In addition some (although not all) investigators have observed an increase in diet-induced thermogenesis in trained animals (10) and humans (11). These observations prompted us to assess whether insulin affects thermogenesis (as reflected by O_2 consumption) in skeletal muscle following exercise. Hindquarters of rats subjected to intense exercise were perfused as before and O_2 consumption was measured. As shown in Table 1-3, O_2 consumption was not increased in control rats by perfusion with increasing concentrations of insulin. Likewise, no increase in O_2 consumption was observed in preparations from exercised rats perfused without added insulin. On the other hand addition of insulin to the perfusion medium in the exercised group caused a 30% increase in O_2 consumption. This effect was

Table 1-3. Oxygen Consumption by the Perfused Rat Hindquarter Following Intense Exercise[a]

	O_2 Consumption (μmol/g/h)		
		Postexercise	
Insulin (μU/ml)	No Exercise	30 minutes	15 minutes
0	24.7 ± 1.9	23.2 ± 0.9	21.2 ± 1.8
75	23.9 ± 1.3	29.7 ± 1.8*+	29.8 ± 1.5*+
20,000	26.5 ± 1.7	32.4 ± 1.9*+	30.0 ± 1.7*+

[a]Results are means ± SE of at least five experiments. The symbols * and + indicate values significantly different from those of the no exercise group and the groups perfused with no added insulin, respectively, $p < .05$. Adapted from Balon and coworkers (9).

present in hindquarters perfused both 30 and 150 minutes after the cessation of exercise and it was as great at physiological (75μU/ml) as at supraphysiological (20,000 μU/ml) insulin concentrations. The basis for the increase in thermogenesis is not known. It correlated poorly with the stimulation of glucose utilization by insulin and it could be only partially accounted for by the energy required for increased glycogen synthesis (9). Possibly alterations in substrate cycling or ion fluxes play a role; however this remains to be determined.

In humans, a situation analogous to that of the perfused hindquarter could occur when an individual raises his plasma insulin level by eating after having exercised. To test this notion normal volunteers were run on a treadmill at 70% of their VO_{2max} for 45 minutes. Approximately 2 hours later, when their VO_2 had returned to baseline values, they received 100 g of glucose by mouth and thermogenesis was assessed over the next 3 hours by indirect calorimetry. On a separate day, on which the subjects did not exercise, the test procedure was repeated. Results for two representative subjects are shown in Table 1-4. At almost all time points after glucose administration the increase in O_2 consumption induced by glucose was greater on the exercise day. Seven patients have been studied to date and for this group the incre-

Table 1-4. Effect of Prior Exercise on Diet-Induced Thermogenesis in Two Representative Subjects[a]

Time after Glucose Administration (minutes):	VO_2 (% of initial value)				
	10	30	60	120	180
T.B. Postexercise	72	55	30	34	17
Control	24	19	26	8	20
J.Y. Postexercise	36	32	29	21	32
Control	15	23	22	3	19

[a]Glucose (100 g) was administered to the postexercise group after VO_2 had returned to resting values. Control values were obtained at the same time on a subsequent day on which the subject had not exercised (Young and coworkers unpublished data).

ment in O_2 consumption induced by glucose over 3 hours is more than twice as great on the exercise day (12).

These data must still be regarded as preliminary; nevertheless when considered in conjunction with the hindquarter studies they suggest that (1) insulin stimulates thermogenesis following intense exercise and (2) a major site at which this occurs is skeletal muscle. The quantitative contribution of this postexercise increase in thermogenesis to the weight loss observed in some subjects who initiate a program of intense endurance exercise remains to be determined. Data reported in this volume by Garrow (Chapter 4) and by Pi-Sunyer suggest that a similar phenomenon may not occur if the exercise is of mild to moderate intensity.

Metabolic and hormonal alterations occur in the postexercise state. The focus of this chapter has been on insulin action in muscle; however, alterations of other hormones and in other tissues, for example, bone, almost certainly occur. Some of these effects appear to be clinically relevant and have led to the recommendation that exercise be used in the treatment or prevention of various disorders. It must be emphasized, however, that the therapeutic use of exercise is still in its infancy and that knowledge of how exercise should be used would benefit greatly from a better understanding of the mechanisms by which it acts.

REFERENCES

1. J. O. Holloszy and F. W. Booth, *Ann. Rev. Physiol.,* **29,** 273 (1976).
2. S. Maehlum, P. Felig, and J. Wahren, *Am. J. Physiol.,* **234,** E255 (1978).
3. E. A. Richter, L. P. Garetto, M. N. Goodman, and N. B. Ruderman: *J. Clin. Invest.,* **69,** 785 (1982).
4. L. P. Garetto, E. A. Richter, M. N. Goodman, and N. B. Ruderman, *Am. J. Physiol.,* **246,** E471 (1984).
5. S. Schneider, L. Amoroso, N. B. Ruderman, and A. Khachadurian, *Diabetologia,* **26,** 355 (1984).
6. G. W. Heath, J. R. Gavin, III, J. M. Hinderliter, J. M. Hagberg, S. A. Bloomfield, and J. O. Holloszy, *J. Appl. Physiol.,* **55(2),** 512 (1983).
7. K. Acheson, E. Jequier, and J Wahren, *J. Clin. Invest.,* **72,** 981 (1983).

8. R. A. DeFronzo, D. Thorin, J. P. Felber, D. C. Simonson, D. Thiebaud, E. Jequier, and A. Golay, *J. Clin. Invest.*, **73,** 633 (1984).
9. T. W. Balon, A. Zorzano, M. N. Goodman, and N. B. Ruderman, *Am. J. Physiol.*, **248,** (1984), in press.
10. M. Gleeson, J. F. Brown, J. J. Waring, and M. J. Stock, *Brit. J. Nutr.*, **47,** 173 (1982).
11. J. Davis, A. R. Tagliaferro, R. Kertzer, T. Gerardo, J. Nichols, and J. Wheeler, *Eur. J. Appl. Physiol. Occup. Physiol.*, **509,** 319 (1983).
12. J. C. Young, J. L. Treadway, and N. B. Ruderman, "Effect of Prior Exercise on Dietary-Induced thermogenesis," in, *Med. Sci. Sports Exerc.*, (1985), in press (abstract).

2

Protein and Amino Acid Metabolism in Relation to Physical Exercise

VERNON R. YOUNG, Ph.D.

Massachusetts Institute of Technology, Cambridge, Massachusetts

There has long been interest in the interrelationships between physical exercise, protein nutrition, and the metabolism of amino acids and proteins. A number of recent reviews have explored, in detail, various aspects of this topic (1–4) and so this short chapter will present overview of some selected areas of current research, giving attention to the question of protein and amino acid requirements in relation to physical exercise. The effects of physical activity on muscle and whole body, and on muscle protein and amino acid metabolism will be considered first. Against this background the possible effects of exercise on the protein and amino acid requirements of the host then can be explored. The literature cited here will not be comprehensive but, where possible, we will refer to review papers to give the interested reader a broader access to the published material.

PROTEIN AND AMINO ACID METABOLISM—MAINLY ANIMAL MODELS

Muscle Protein Metabolism

It is important to examine first how exercise affects protein and amino acid metabolism in the tissues most immediately involved in exercise, namely the skeletal musculature. It is particularly relevant to consider this problem because this tissue plays a quantitatively significant role in whole body protein metabolism (5) and an effect of exercise on muscles, therefore, may determine the status of protein and amino acid metabolism in the body as a whole.

As summarized in Table 2-1, studies from our laboratories (7,8,12,13) and those of other investigators (9–11,14,15) show that rates of whole body protein synthesis and breakdown under steady state conditions in the healthy adult approximate about 4 g protein/kg/day. Although the contributions of different tissues to protein turnover in the whole body cannot be stated with precision, Lobley and coworkers (16) estimate that in most species muscle accounts for between 15 and 20%. For man the estimates are limited, but we (17) and Tomas and coworkers (18) have estimated that muscle protein turnover accounts for about 1 g protein/kg/day or approximately 25–30% of whole body protein turnover. However, from measurements of the incorporation of 1-^{13}C-leucine into muscle proteins Rennie and coworkers (15) concluded that muscle accounted for more than 50% of the turn-

Table 2-1. Summary of Some Estimates of Whole Body Protein Synthesis in Normal Adult Man[a]

Authors	Tracer Used	Synthesis Rate (g protein/kg/day)
Steffee et al. (7)	^{15}N-glycine	3.0 ± 0.13[b]
Winterer et al. (8)	^{15}N-glycine	3.3 ± 0.15
Fern et al. (9)	^{15}N-glycine	4.0 ± 0.1
Fern et al. (10)	^{15}N-glycine	4.1 ± 0.07
Birkhahn et al. (11)	^{15}N-glycine	3.1 ± 0.37
Motil et al. (12)	^{13}C-leucine	4.3 ± 0.11
Motil et al. (13)	^{13}C-leucine	5.5 ± 0.32
Clugston and Garlick (14)	^{13}C-leucine	4.37 ± 0.42
Rennie et al. (15)	^{13}C-leucine	6.07 ± 0.45

[a]Taken from part of Table 2 of Waterlow (6), where further details concerning the tracer method used in each study are given.
[b]Mean ± SEM.

over of proteins in the whole body of normal, fed adults. In spite of these differing estimates it is clear that muscle accounts for a significant component of total body protein turnover and it is relevant, therefore, to ask the question of what happens to protein synthesis and breakdown in muscles during exercise.

This subject has been reviewed recently (1,3) but some general comments can be made. First, in reference to endurance-type exercise the rate of ^{14}C-labeled amino acid incorporation by the perfused hindquarter in rats and by isolated polyribosomes in vitro is depressed with a single acute bout of exercise (Table 2-2)(19) and this decline can be even greater if the exercise continues to exhaustion (20). Similarly, during maximal isometric contraction rates of protein synthesis are markedly inhibited, with a return to initial resting rates during the recovery period (Table 2-3) (21). Thus, although it is difficult to draw an entirely clear picture of the effects of exercise on skeletal muscle protein synthesis in laboratory animals, particularly because of possible differences in the response of different muscles and fiber types, and in the intensity and duration of the exercise studied, it seems reasonable to conclude that there is a decline in protein synthesis during the period of exercise.

Table 2-2. Effects of an Acute Bout of Exercise (1 h swim) on Protein Synthesis and Breakdown Using a Perfused Hemicorpus Preparation and Muscle Polyribosomes[a]

	Synthesis		
Group	^{3}H-Tyrosine Incorporation[b] (nmole/hour/mg) protein)	^{14}C-Leucine Incorporation by Polyribosomes (pmole/min/mg RNA)	Breakdown Rate[c]
Rested	0.32	3.4	8.9
Exercised	0.26	2.5	13.8

[a]Summarized from Dohm *et al.* (19).
[b]Soluble protein fraction of perfused muscle.
[c]μmol tyrosine release/hour per hemicorpus.

Table 2-3. Protein Synthesis and Degradation in Perfused Hind Limb Muscles[a]

	Protein Synthesis[b]		
State	TA	Gastroc	MH Release[c]
Resting	140	139	15.5
Contracting	31	5	3.6

[a]Summarized from Bylund-Fellenius et al. (21).
[b]nmol phe/g.
[c]pmol/min/g (N^{τ}-methylhistidine).

It is also relevant to record that there also appears to be a reduced rate of liver protein synthesis in exercising rats (3) and that the depression is greatest with exhaustive exercise (3). Furthermore, liver protein degradation appears to be elevated (22,23).

Whether exercise brings about a change in the rate of muscle protein degradation is less certain, as shown, for example, by the differences in results summarized in Tables 2-2 and 2-3. Thus, Dohm and coworkers (19) assessed protein muscle degradation in a perfused hind limb quarter by measurement of tyrosine release, as well as by measurement of N^{τ}-methylhistidine (Mehis) excretion during a strenuous bout of exercise in rats (24). Both measures of muscle protein degradation appeared to demonstrate an elevation in protein breakdown with exercise. In contrast, Bylund-Fellenius and coworkers (21) (see Table 2-3) observed a reduction in the rate of release of Mehis from contracting muscle, concommitant with a reduced free content of this compound in muscle compared with the resting condition. Therefore, their data suggest, at least, that myofibrillar protein degradation during muscle contraction may be reduced.

The effects of exercise on rates of protein synthesis and breakdown in human muscles remain to be explored critically, but some limited observations will be discussed below.

Amino Acid Metabolism

Changes in rates of protein synthesis, and possibly in the rate of breakdown, in muscles and other tissues are associated with alterations in the free amino acid content of plasma, muscle, and liver. Thus, for example, Dohm and coworkers (3) report increases in the whole body tyrosine level after exhaustive exercise and increases in the concentration of leucine in plasma, liver, and muscle in rats that swim for 1–2 hours or run to exhaustion (25). Such changes might account for, or be due to, alterations in the rates of oxidation of amino acids. Thus, studies show, for example, increased leucine oxidation in exercised rats (26,27). Furthermore, muscle homogenates from trained rats show an enhanced capacity to oxidize this amino acid (28) and there is a relationship between the intensity of exercise and leucine oxidation in rats (26) as well as in man (29). In association with such changes in amino acid oxidation there is a rise in the rate of alanine release from muscle during exercise.

In summary, based on studies in rats, endurance-type exercise appears to result in a depression in muscle protein synthesis and in increased rates of amino acid oxidation, especially with respect to the branched chain amino acid, leucine. The human relevance of these findings will be considered shortly.

More Chronic Exercise

The effects of chronic exercise on muscle protein metabolism have been explored using various approaches and models. Thus, changes in muscle protein metabolism that occur during hypertrophy of muscles induced by increased work loads have received attention and this topic has been reviewed earlier by Millward (30). The different models have advantages and limitations in relation to an understanding of the physiology of exercise and protein metabolism but collectively the available data help identify further the basic responses of protein metabolism in muscle to altered levels and types of physical activity.

A list of results of some studies, carried out with these various models that result in muscular hypertrophy, concerned with various aspects of muscle protein metabolism and altered activity patterns is given in Table 2-4. A number of the studies reveal that amino acid transport is enhanced with increased work, as is the rate of incorporation of labeled amino acids into mixed proteins and sarcoplasmic and fibrillar protein fractions. Furthermore, there are changes in the metabolism and content of nucleic acids (RNA and DNA) that favor increased rates of protein synthesis and growth of muscle with higher work loads. From this summary it appears that there is a series of changes in nucleic acid metabolism and in the protein synthetic machinery of muscle cells that are regulated coordinately following an alteration

Table 2-4. Some Observations Relating to Protein Synthesis During Muscular Hypertrophy

Process (model)	Authors
Amino Acid Transport	
AIB accumulation (tetonomy)	Goldberg et al. (31)
AIB accumulation (stimulation in vitro)	Goldberg et al. (31)
AIB accumulation (denervation, diaphragm)	Buse et al. (32)
Protein Synthesis (in vitro, in vivo)	
^{14}C-amino acid incorporation	Laurent and Sparrow (33)
^{14}C-amino acid incorporation	Goldberg et al. (34)
^{14}C-amino acid incorporation	Laurent et al. (35)
Ribosome activity	Turner and Manchester (36)
Cell-sap activity	Turner and Manchester (36)
Microsomal activity	Hamosh et al. (37)
Nucleic acid	
RNA plymerase	Sobel and Kaufman (38)
^{3}H-thymidine into DNA	Goldbeg et al. (34)
DNA, RNA content	Various authors

in the work load imposed upon this organ. However, the initial metabolic events and specific changes that lead to this complex set of alterations in muscle protein metabolism remain to be determined.

It must also be pointed out that not only does intracellular protein synthesis increase when muscle is stimulated to become hypertrophic as a result of increased work loads, but the content and rate of collagen synthesis and activity of protocollagen proline-hydroxylase (39) are also increased. However, Laurent and coworkers (40) suggest that the increase in collagen synthesis accounts for only a small percentage of the total increase in protein synthesis in muscles undergoing stretch-induced hypertrophy.

Changes in protein synthesis may also be accompanied by alterations in the rate of protein breakdown and in Table 2-5 a summary is given of the conclusions by various authors about the effects of exercise on protein breakdown. Again, as discussed above for the case of acute exercise, it is evident that there is little consistency among the various studies; some have con-

Table 2-5. Some Observations on the Effects of Exercise on Protein Breakdown

Muscle and Condition	Response of Breakdown	Authors
Soleus-tetonomy	Reduced[a]	Goldberg (41)
Soleus-stimulated, stretched	Reduced[a]	Goldberg (42)
EDL-immobilized, lengthened	Increased[b]	Goldspink (43)
EDL-denervated, stretched	Increased[b]	Goldspink (44)
Diaphragm-denervated	Increased[a]	Turner and Garlick (45)
ALD (weighting)	No change[a]	Laurent and Sparrow (33)
ALD (weighting)	Increased[a]	Laurent et al. (35)

[a]In vivo measurement.
[b]In vitro measurement.

cluded that breakdown does not change, others that it is decreased, and still others that it is increased. The reasons for these variable conclusions may relate to the use of different models as well as to the different methods used to estimate actual breakdown rates. The latter are not readily determined with accuracy or precision. Using a technique based on a continuous infusion of labeled amino acids in vivo, Turner and Garlick (45) and Laurent and coworkers (35) have concluded that rates of protein synthesis and breakdown both increase during muscular hypertrophy.

Based on their work on stretch-induced hypertrophy, Laurent and Millward (46) found in the anterior latissimus dorsi (ALD) muscles of the fully grown fowl (*Gallus domesticus*) that rates of muscle protein synthesis and breakdown are increased rapidly and that this increase was sustained until growth of the ALD muscle had been achieved. At this time these rates returned to values obtained before treatment (weighting of the wing) was introduced. It appears that there was a considerable "wasteage" of protein synthesis or increased protein turnover, which may be due to a remodeling of muscle associated with growth. An increased lysosomal enzyme activity in muscle of mice with training (47) is compatible with higher rates of muscle protein breakdown during or immediately following increased exercise.

Based on the foregoing a summary picture is presented in Figure 2-1 illustrating the multiple points at which chronic exercise has been shown to affect amino acid and protein metabolism in muscle cells.

Some Comments on Mechanisms

Before considering the effects of exercise on protein and amino acid in humans, it is worth raising the question of the signals that initiate changes in protein metabolism leading to hypertrophy or altered enzyme profiles in exercised muscles. These signals may include neutrotophic factors, passive stretch, contractile activity, and increased tension (48). All of these signals may play a role and the importance of stretch, both active and pas-

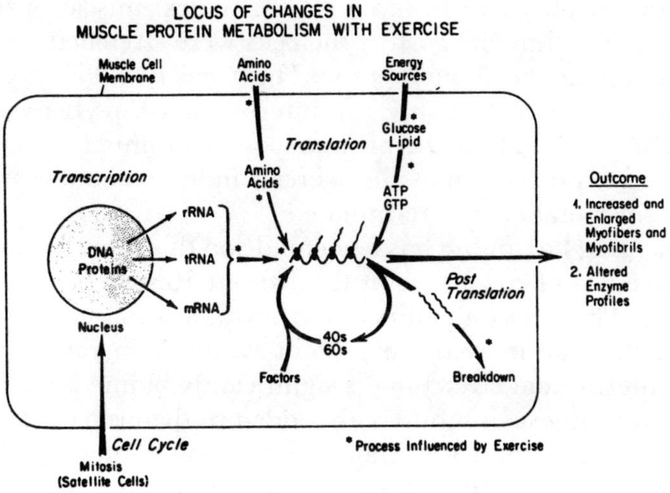

Figure 2-1. Schematic outline of the major phases of amino acid utilization and protein turnover (synthesis and breakdown) in the muscle cell and points at which exercise has been shown to effect changes in the rate and pattern of protein synthesis and content.

sive, as a key factor is now quite clear. This conclusion is strengthened by the elegant study of Vandenburgh and Kaufman (49) as summarized in Table 2-6. Amino acid transport, rates of total and myofibrillar protein synthesis, and the protein content

Table 2-6. Effect of a 10.8% Mechanical Stretch of Embryonic Chicken Skeletal Myotubes in Culture[a]

Parameter	Effect of Stretch (% Change)
AIB accumulation	+30
^{14}C-leu incorporation:	
Total protein	+14
Myosin HC	+16
Protein:	
Total	+ 8.7
Myosin HC	+14.7

[a]Summarized from Vandenburgh and Kaufman (49).

of myotubes, obtained from embryonic chick muscle, grown in culture, were stimulated when the cells were stretched by growing them on an elastic membrane. However, it will be necessary to explore more thoroughly the interrelationships between the basic structural and biochemical responses of muscle to exercise to determine precisely how the exercise-induced changes in muscle protein metabolism are initiated.

An exciting beginning has been made on this topic by the studies of Reeds and coworkers at the Rowett Research Institute in Scotland. These investigators have shown, as summarized in Table 2-7, that the increase in protein synthesis in rabbit muscle due to intermittent stretching is significantly blunted when prostaglandin synthesis inhibitors are added to the preparation (50). Furthermore, as shown in Table 2-8, in a subsequent study they related the stimulation of protein synthesis with intermittent stretching to an increased release of PGF_2 (51). Because phospholipase is associated with the cell membrane, it is possible that stretching causes an activation of the enzyme, resulting in an increase in the liberation of arachidonic acid from phospholipid, leading to an increased conversion of this essential fatty acid to its eicosanoid products, including the prostaglandins, thromboxanes, and leukotrienes (52).

The further possible involvement of eicosanoids in the exercise-

Table 2-7. Effect of Inhibitors of Prostaglandin Synthesis on Stretch-induced Muscle Protein Synthesis[a]

	Protein Synthesis (%/day)	
	Constant Tension	Intermittent Stretching
Control	2.47	5.21
Control + indomethacin	2.85	3.01*
Control	2.2	4.1
Control + meclofenamate	1.9	2.7*

[a]Summarized from Smith et al. (50).

Table 2-8. Effect of Intermittent Stretching on Protein Synthesis and PGF_2 Release[a]

Condition	Protein Synthesis (%/day)	PGF_2 Release (pg/90 min/mg)
Constant tension	2.3	10.1
Constant tension + indomthacin	2.1	9.7
Intermittent tension	3.4	22.6
Intermittent tension + indomethacin	2.1	9.6

[a]Palmer et al. (51).

induced alterations of protein and amino acid metabolism is suggested by the study of Cannon and Kluger (53). These workers found that a 1 hour exercise at 60% VO_{2max} on a bicycle ergometer in healthy human volunteers brought about an increased release of endogenous pyrogen (presumably interleukin-1(IL-1)) from mononuclear leukocytes. Among the many actions of IL-1 (54) is its ability to induce muscle protein breakdown, possibly via a stimulation in the rate of formation of PGE_2 (55).

From these recent observations it appears that the eicosanoids, including the prostaglandins, might serve as mediators for the exercise-induced alterations in protein and amino acid metabolism. Clearly, this represents an area for further important and exciting research, particularly since this area is relevant not only to the question of exercise but to growth, maturation, and metabolism of muscles in general.

PROTEIN AND AMINO ACID METABOLISM—HUMAN SUBJECTS

The impact of exercise on muscle and body protein metabolism in man has not been explored to the depth that has been achieved in animal models. However, it is possible to draw some general comparisons between the observations discussed above and the metabolic responses to exercise in human volunteers.

First, a number of groups of investigators have explored the effect of exercise on whole body protein turnover and amino acid kinetics, using a constant isotope-tracer infusion approach. In all of these studies (56–59) the incorporation of leucine into whole body proteins has been found to be decreased during exercise (Table 2-9). However, the effects of exercise on protein degradation are less clear. Dohm and coworkers (24), as shown in Table 2-10, reported an increased rate of excretion of Mehis with exercise in humans, implying an increased rate of myofibrillar protein breakdown. Others, however, found no change (60) or a decrease (56,61). Furthermore, results from isotopic studies of whole body protein breakdown are equally variable; some have found increased rates (56,57), others no change (62), and we (59) observed a decrease during exercise. Thus, the effects of exercise on muscle and whole body protein turnover in man remain to be clarified.

However, it can be concluded, as we (59) (Table 2-9) and others have shown, that the rate of leucine oxidation is significantly enhanced during exercise in humans. Furthermore, the in-

Table 2-9. Parameters of Whole Body Leucine Kinetics in Subjects at Rest and During 2 Hours of Exercise at 55% VO_{2max}[a]

Parameters	Condition		p
	Rest	Exercise	
Leucine flux	120.4 + 6.2(15)[b]	97.0 ± 7.13(15)	<.001
Leucine oxidation	14.8 + 1.3(8)	46.1 ± 9.7(8)	<.01
Leucine incorporation into protein	113.2 + 5.4(8)	58.2 ± 9.5(8)	<.01

[a]Summarized from Evans et al. (59).
[b]Values are μmole/kg/hour. Mean ± SEM. Number of subjects in parentheses.

Table 2-10. Effect of an Exercise Bout on Urea and N^{τ}-Methylhistidine (MH) Excretion in Human Subjects[a]

	Urea	MH
Runners		
Preexercise	406[b]	286[c]
Postexercise	730*	514*
Weightlifters		
Preexercise	654	588
Postexercise	864	678

[a]Summarized from Dohm et al. (24).
[b]mmol/day.
[c]μmol/day.

creased rate of leucine oxidation is related to the intensity of the exercise, although the effect of exercise on leucine oxidation might be modulated by the current nutritional status of the host (62).

The increased rate of leucine oxidation is consistent with the rise in blood urea (63), increased sweat urea excretion (2), and increased urinary nitrogen output (2,4,64) with exercise in human subjects. It is unclear, however, whether the additional urea is produced mainly during or after the exercise bout, and this requires further exploration. Furthermore, the extent to which changes in leucine oxidation are indicative of alterations in the oxidation of other amino acids deserves additional study. Indeed, the effects of exercise on the metabolic fate of the specific, nutritionally indispensable (essential) amino acids, and on the dispensable (nonessential) amino acids, as well as on the interrelationships between these classes of amino acid, represent an area of investigation for those concerned with defining more completely the impact of exercise on protein and amino acid metabolism in human subjects.

An exciting point that might be made here, in relation to the changes in amino acid oxidation mentioned above, concerns the possible contribution of these energy yielding substrates to overall energy needs of the exercising subject. Thus, using our data for leucine oxidation it would appear, as summarized in Table

Table 2-11. Contribution of Protein Oxidation[a] to Total Energy Expenditure[b] (%) at Rest and During 2 Hours of Exercise at 55% VO_{2max}[c]

Subjects	No.	Preexercise	During exercise
Untrained	3	14.1	4.8
Trained	5	12.2	2.9

[a]Based upon leucine content in whole body protein of 590 μmol/kg/hour (preexercise) and 46.1 μmol/kg/hour (during exercise).
[b]Total energy expenditure derived from indirect calorimetry using measured values of VO_2 and R during a 2 hour period.
[c]Data of Evans et al. (59).

2-11, that the oxidation of protein would account for less than about 5% of energy expenditure during exercise. Dohm and coworkers (3) have made equivalent calculations for exercising rats and estimate that possibly as much as 20–25% of the extra energy expenditure might be contributed by the complete oxidation of amino acids released from proteins. However, as indicated above, the proportionate contribution made by total amino acid catabolism to the total energy expenditure in human subjects may actually be lower during exercise than at rest. Hence, our observations are entirely consistent with the notion that carbohydrate- and lipid-derived fuels are the major substrates for enhanced oxidative catabolism during exercise.

In summary, some general statements are made in Table 2-12 concerning effects of vigorous exercise on human protein and amino acid metabolism. At this point, it is appropriate to con-

Table 2-12. Protein Metabolism in Endurance Exercise: Summary of Observations

Protein synthesis is *decreased.*
Protein degradation is decreased/increased?
Leucine oxidation is increased.
Oxidation of other indispensable amino acids requires study.
Gluconeogenesis is *increased* (see Ref. 3 for review).

sider the subject of exercise with reference to the nutrition requirements for protein and indispensable amino acids.

PROTEIN AND AMINO ACID REQUIREMENTS IN RELATION TO EXERCISE

A Metabolic View

Although the increase in leucine oxidation during exercise discussed above is of relatively minor importance in relation to overall aspects of energy expenditure, the status of leucine oxidation may have more important implications with respect to the amino acid and N economy of the host. Furthermore, because urea accounts for the major proportion of total urinary N excretion in well-nourished subjects, changes in urea production and excretion with exercise should reflect changes in body N balance. Indeed, there is evidence that the latter becomes more negative when moderate exercise is required in healthy men receiving a generous intake of protein and adequate energy (65,66) (Figure 2-2). Hence, it can be suggested that moderate to heavy exercise might increase the requirement for total N, at least during the initial weeks of a program of moderate physical activity. This increased requirement appears even more likely if the increased losses of N via sweat are also taken into account (2).

There have been an insufficient number of studies to examine this issue in much greater depth but we have shown, as depicted in Figure 2-3, that a period of training of isometric exercise in healthy adult men results in a reduction in body potassium, and probably body cell mass, when the test subjects consumed a diet approximating the 1973 FAO/WHO (68) dietary protein allowance (0.6 g protein/kg/day). In contrast, these changes did not occur when subjects were first adapted to a diet providing a more generous intake of 1 g egg protein/kg/day (67). Furthermore, a change in protein requirement as a consequence of exercise is also suggested by the data of Yoshimura and coworkers (69). These investigators have shown that during training to strenuous physical exercise, the content of hemoglobin in circulating blood

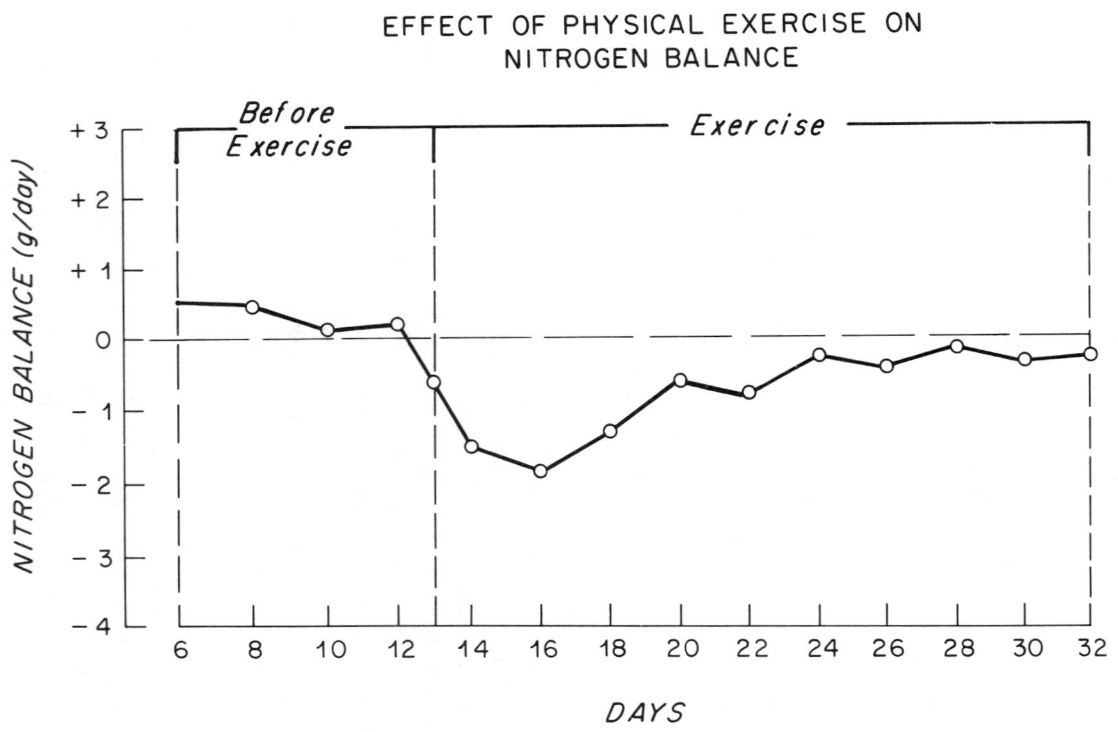

Figure 2-2. Mean nitrogen balance for 12 healthy young men before and during a 3 week period of increased physical activity (9.9 Kcal/minute for 6 of each 20 minute periods per day). Subjects received 1 g protein/kg/day (35% from animal origin). Drawn from Gontzea and coworkers (65).

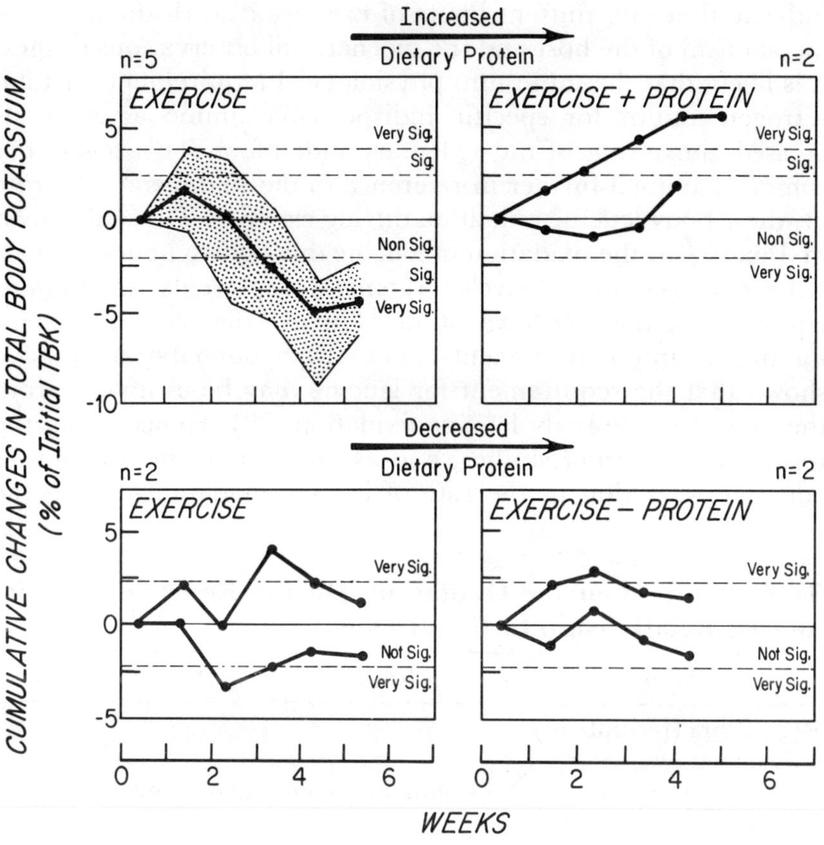

Figure 2-3. Weekly mean cumulative changes in total body potassium (TBK) in young men receiving 0.5 or 1.0 g egg protein/kg/day while performing a 75 minute isometric exercise program daily for 4 to 6 weeks. Drawn from Torun and coworkers (67).

decreased when subjects received a diet containing about 1.3 to 1.5 g protein/kg/day, but that this did not occur when the level of protein intake was 2.5 g/kg/day. These observations were interpreted to indicate that a high intake of protein is required during the course of physical training (69).

In spite of the early work suggesting the lack of an effect of physical exercise per se on the minimum physiologic protein requirement of the host, the more recent studies referred to here indicate that intermittent bouts of exercise disturb the nitrogen metabolism of the host and the biochemical observations suggest it is likely that the minimum physiological requirement for total nitrogen and/or for specific indispensable amino acids is increased above that of the sedentary individual. This possibility can be examined further in reference to the findings on the rate of whole body leucine oxidation during exercise. Thus, as shown in Table 2-13, the oxidation of leucine during two hours of moderate exercise on a bicycle ergometer represents an amount equivalent to the *upper range* of the estimated dietary requirement for this amino acid. Recent studies from our laboratory have shown that the requirement for leucine may be estimated from the rate of whole body leucine oxidation (70). Hence, from the results of our recent studies, and assuming that there is not an adaptive reduction in the rate of leucine oxidation during the

Table 2-13. Leucine Oxidation[a] During Rest and Exercise and Its Relationship to Requirement

Status	Rate	Total Quantity
Rest: 2 hrs (recumbent)		
Leucine oxidation	14.8μmol/kg/hour	2087 μmol = 274 mg
Leucine[b] Requirement	14.0 mg/kg/day	987 mg
Oxidation: Percent of requirement		28
Exercise: 2 hrs (55% VO_{2max})		
Leucine oxidation	46.1μmol/kg/hour	6500 μmol = 853 mg
Leucine[b] requirement		987 mg
Oxidation: Percent of requirement		86

[a]Untrained subjects (mean weight 70.5 kg). Based on Evans et al. (59).
[b]FAO/WHO (68).

postexercise period in comparison with that rate for nonexercised subjects, the minimum physiological requirement for this amino acid would be predicted to be higher for physically active than for sedentary subjects. Of course, another possibility to be considered in the interpretation of these data is that the rate of leucine oxidation during exercise may be determined, in part, by the previous dietary intake level of leucine. Hence, it is possible that subjects who had been adapted to a lower protein or essential amino acid intake may not show the marked increase in leucine oxidation that was observed in our subjects who had received a generous protein intake for a number of days prior to the exercise test. Furthermore, leucine oxidation rates, especially during the absorptive phases of amino acid metabolism, fall when the intake of dietary leucine or protein is lowered (70). Therefore, it would also be of interest to determine whether a period of exercise induces a significant increase in leucine oxidation in subjects previously adapted to a diet that provides leucine at levels approximating current estimates of the requirement for this amino acid. If an increase in leucine oxidation was observed in trained subjects under these dietary conditions, it would provide convincing evidence that the minimum physiological requirement for this amino acid is determined, in part, by physical activity per se.

Finally, it is important to emphasize that the metabolism of leucine is closely associated with the skeletal muscles. Although it is tempting to interpret a change in leucine oxidation during exercise as indicative of a general increase in the oxidation of indispensable (essential) amino acids, it will be important to determine directly whether exercise alters significantly the rate of oxidation of amino acids that are catabolized predominantly in the liver, such as lysine, and tyrosine.

Results of N Balance Studies

Although the minimum physiological requirement for leucine, for example, might be increased as discussed above, the minimum requirements for both indispensable amino acids and total protein in adults are less than the usual dietary intake levels of most free-living healthy individuals. Hence, it is important to determine whether exercise causes a change in nitrogen balance and overall utilization of dietary nitrogen (protein) when the dietary supply of protein corresponds more closely to usual levels of intake. Table 2-14 presents a summary of a number of studies in which the protein intake approached or exceeded these levels; the overall results indicate that body protein balance is maintained with exercise under these conditions involving generous protein intakes.

Therefore, from this set of observations it is reasonable to conclude that at intakes of protein amounting to about 1–1.5g/kg body weight/day, or approximately 75–100g daily, the total nitrogen and amino acid intake is sufficient to support the needs

Table 2-14. Nitrogen Balance Studies Concerning Dietary Protein Requirements for Exercise

Investigators	Exercise Period	Protein Intake (g/kg/day)	Nitrogen Balance Status
Gontzea et al. (65,66)	4 days	1.0	Negative
	4 days	1.5	Positive
	3 weeks	1.0	Initially negative, approached equilibrium after 2-3 weeks
Consolazio et al. (71)	40 days	1.4	Positive
	40 days	2.4	More positive than for lower protein group
Marable et al. (72)	11 days	2.0	Decrease in urinary N excretion during last 14 days for both groups when compared to controls
Celejowa and Homa (73)	11 days	2.0	Slightly positive
Torun et al. (67)	42 days	1.0	Maintained body potassium

for all exercises. On this basis the usual diet, supplying approximately 15–17% of the total energy as protein, should be adequate. Thus, there would be little rationale for either taking or recommending use of protein supplements or unusually generous amounts of high protein foods (see also 4,74, 75). The same conclusions also apply to the use of vitamin or mineral supplements (76).

REFERENCES

1. V. R. Young and B. Torun, "Physical Activity: Impact on Protein and Amino Acid Metabolism and Implications for Nutritional Requirements," in *Nutrition in Health and Disease and International Development.* Alan R. Liss, New York, 1981, pp. 57–85.
2. P. W. R. Leman and F. T. Nagle, *Med. Sci. Sports Exercise,* **13,** 141 (1981).
3. G. L. Dohm, G. J. Kasperek, E. B. Tapscott, and H. A. Barakat, *Fed. Proc.* **44,** 348 (1985).
4. G. L. Dohm, *Clinics Sports Med.,* **3,** 595 (1984).
5. V. R. Young, "Role of Skeletal and Cardiac Muscle in the Regulation of Body Protein Metabolism," in H. N. Munro, Ed., *Mammalian Protein Metabolism* Vol. 4, Academic, New York, 1970.
6. J. C. Waterlow, *Quart. J. Exptl. Physiol.,* **69,** 409 (1984).
7. W. P. Steffee, R. S. Goldsmith, P. B. Pencharz, N. S. Scrimshaw, and V. R. Young, *Metabolism,* **25,** 281 (1976).
8. J. C. Winterer, W. P. Steffe, W. D. A. Perera, R. Uauy, N. S. Scrimshaw, and V. R. Young, *Exptl. Gerontol.,* **11,** 79 (1976).
9. E. B. Fern, P. J. Garlick, M. A. McNurlan, and J. C. Waterlow, *Clin. Sci.,* **61,** 217 (1981).
10. E. B. Fern, P. J. Garlick, H. Sheppard, and M. Fern, *Human Nutrition: Clinical Nutrition,* **38C,** 63 (1984).
11. R. H. Birkhahn, C. L. Long, D. Fitkin, M. Jeevanandan, and W. S. Blakemore, *Am. J. Physiol.,* **241,** E67 (1981).
12. K. J. Motil, D. M. Bier, D. E. Matthews, J. F. Burke, and V. R. Young, *Metabolism,* **30,** 783 (1981).
13. K. J. Motil, D. E. Matthews, D. M. Bier, J. F. Burke, H. N. Munro, and V. R. Young, *Am. J. Physiol.,* **240,** E712 (1981).
14. G. Clugston and P. J. Garlick, *Human Nutrition: Clinical Nutrition,* **36C,** 57 (1982).
15. M. J. Rennie, R. H. T. Edwards, D. Halliday, D. E. Matthews, S. L. Wolman, and D. J. Millward, *Clin. Sci.,* **63,** 519 (1982).
16. G. E. Lobley, V. Milne, J. M. Lovie, P. J. Reeds, and K. Pennie, *Brit. J. Nutr.,* **43,** 491 (1980).

17. R. Uauy, J. C. Winterer, C. Bilmazes, L. N. Haverberg, N. S. Scrimshaw, H. N. Munro, and V. R. Young, *J. Gerontol.*, **33,** 663 (1978).
18. F. M. Tomas, F. J. Ballard, and L. M. Pope, *Clin. Sci.*, **56,** 341 (1979).
19. G. L. Dohm, G. J. Kosparek, E. B. Tapscott, and G. R. Beecher, *Biochem. J.*, **188,** 255 (1980).
20. G. L. Dohm, E. B. Tapscott, H. A. Barakat, and G. J. Kasperek, *Biochem. Med.*, **27,** 367 (1982).
21. A. C. Bylund-Fellenius, K. M. Ojama, K. E. Flaim, J. B. Li, S. J. Wassner, and L. S. Jefferson, Protein synthesis versus energy state in contracting muscles of perfused rat hind limb. (1984).
22. G. J. Kasperek, G. L. Dohm, H. A. Barakat, P. H. Strausbauch, D. W. Barnes, R. D. Snider, *Biochem. J.*, **202,** 281 (1982).
23. G. J. Kasperek, G. L. Dohm, E. B. Tapscott, and T. Powell, *Proc. Soc. Exp. Biol. Med.*, **164,** 430 (1980).
24. G. L. Dohm, R. T. Williams, G. J. Kasperek, and A. M. van Rij, *J. Appl. Physiol. Respirat. Environ. Exercise. Physiol.*, **52,** (1982).
25. G. L. Dohm, G. R. Beecker, R. O. Warren, and R. T. Williams, *J. Appl. Physiol. Respirat. Environ. Exercise Physiol.*, **50,** 41 (1981).
26. T. P. White and G. A. Brooks, *Am. J. Physiol.*, **240,** E155 (1981).
27. P. W. R. Leman, F. J. Nagle, J. P. Mullin and N. J. Benevenga, *J. Appl. Physiol. Respir. Environ. Exercise Physiol.*, **53,** 947 (1983).
28. G. L. Dohm, A. L. Hecker, W. S. Brown, G. J. Klain, F. R. Puente, E. W. Askew, and G. R. Beecker, *Biochem. J.*, **164,** 705 (1977).
29. D. J. Millward, C. T. M. Davies, D. Halliday, S. L. Wolman, D. Matthews, and M. Rennie, *Fed. Proc.*, **41,** 2686 (1982).
30. D. J. Millward, "Protein Turnover in Skeletal and Cardiac Muscle during Normal Growth and Hypertrophy," in K. Wildenthal, Ed., *Degradative Processes in Heart and Skeletal Muscles,* Elsevier/North Holland, Amsterdam, 1980, p. 161.
31. A. L. Goldberg, C. M. Jablecki, and J. B. Li, *Ann. N.Y. Acad. Sci.*, **228,** 190 (1974).
32. M. G. Buse, J. McMaster, and J. Buse, *Metab.*, **14,** 1220 (1975).
33. G. J. Laurent and M. P. Sparrow, *Growth,* **41,** 249 (1977).
34. A. L. Goldberg, J. D. Etlinger, D. F. Goldspink, and C. Jablecki, *Med. Sci. Sports,* **7,** 185 (1975).
35. G. J. Laurent, M. P. Sparrow, and D. J. Millward, *Biochem. J.*, **176,** 407 (1978).
36. L. V. Turner and K. L. Manchester, *Biochim. Biophys. Acta,* **299,** 612 (1973).
37. M. Homosh, M. Lesch, J. Baron, and S. Kaufman, *Science,* **157,** 935 (1967).
38. B. E. Sobel and S. Kaufman, *Arch. Biochem. Biophys.*, **137,** 469 (1970).
39. H. Turto, S. Lindy, and J. Holme, *Am. J. Physiol.*, **226,** 63 (1974).
40. G. J. Laurent, M. P. Sparrow, P. C. Bates, and D. J. Millward, *Biochem. J.*, **176,** 419 (1978).
41. A. L. Goldberg, *J. Biol. Chem.*, **244,** 3217 (1969).
42. A. L. Goldberg, *Diabetes,* **28** (supplement), 18 (1979).
43. D. F. Goldspink, *J. Physiol.*, **264,** 267 (1977).

44. D. F. Goldspink, *Biochem. J.*, **174,** 595 (1978).
45. L. V. Turner, and P. J. Garlick, *Biochem. Biophys. Acta,* **349,** 109 (1974).
46. G. J. Laurent and D. J. Millward, *Fed. Proc.*, (1979).
47. L. Pilstrom, V. Vihko, E. Astrom, and A. V. Arstila, *Acta Physiol. Scand.*, **104,** 217 (1978).
48. V. R. Young, "Skeletal Muscle and Whole Body Protein Metabolism in Relation to Exercise," in J. Poortmans and G. Miset, Eds., *Biochemistry of Exercise: Exercise and Hormone Regulations,* University Park Press, Baltimore, 1981, p. 59.
49. H. Vandenburgh and S. Kaufman, *Science,* **203,** 265 (1979).
50. R. H. Smith, R. M. Palmer, and P. J. Reeds, *Biochem. J.*, **214,** 153 (1983).
51. R. M. Palmer, P. J. Reeds, T. Atkinson, and R. H. Smith, *Biochem. J.*, **214,** 1011 (1983).
52. A. M. Lefer, *Fed. Proc.*, **44,** 275 (1985).
53. J. C. Canon and M. J. Kluger, *Science,* **220,** 617 (1983).
54. C. A. Dinarello, *New Engl. J. Med.*, **311,** 1413 (1984).
55. V. Baracos, H. P. Rodemann, C. A. Dinarello, and A. L. Goldberg, *New Engl. J. Med.*, **308,** 553 (1983).
56. M. J. Rennie, R. H. T. Edwards, S. Krywawych, C. T. M. Davies, D. Halliday, J. C. Waterlow, and D. J. Millward, *Clin. Sci.*, **61,** 627 (1981).
57. R. R. Wolfe, R. D. Goodenough, M. H. Wolfe, G. T. Royle, and E. R. Nadel, *J. Appl. Physiol. Respir. Environ. Exercise. Physiol.*, **52,** 458 (1981).
58. S. A. Hagg, E. L. Morse, and S. A. Adibi, *Am. J. Physiol.*, **242,** E407 (1982).
59. W. J. Evans, E. D. Wright, S. D. Phinney, D. E. Matthews, D. M. Bier, and V. R. Young, *Med. Sci. Sports Exercise,* (1985) (in press).
60. J. Decombaz, P. Reinhardt, K. Anantharaman, G. van Glutz, and J. R. Poortmans, *Europ. J. Appl. Physiol.*, **41,** 61 (1979).
61. E. Rodha and S. P. Bessman, *Biochem. Med.*, **29,** 96 (1983).
62. M. J. Rennie, D. Halliday, C. T. M. Davies, R. H. T. Edwards, S. Krywawych D. J. Millward, and D. E. Matthews, "Exercise Induced Increase in Leucine Oxidation in Man and the Effect of Glucose," in M. Walser and J. R. Williamson, Eds., *Metabolism and Clinical Implications of Branched Chain Amino Acid Ketoacids,* Elsvier/North Holland, Amsterdam, 1981, pp. 361–366.
63. P. W. R. Leman and J. P. Mullin, *J. Appl. Physiol. Respirat. Environ. Exercise Physiol.*, **48,** 624 (1980).
64. H. E. Refsum and S. B. Stromme, *Scand. J. Clin. Lab. Invest.*, **33,** 247 (1974).
65. I. Gontzea, R. Sutzescu, and S. Dumitrache, *Nutr. Rept. Intl.*, **11,** 231 (1975).
66. I. Gontzea, P. Sutzescu, and S. Dumitrache, *Nutr. Rept. Intl.*, **10,** 35 (1974).
67. B. Torun, N. S. Scrimshaw, and V. R. Young, *Am. J. Clin. Nutr.*, **30,** 1983 (1977).
68. FAO/WHO, "Energy and Protein Requirements," *World Health Organization (WHO) Tech. Rept. Ser. No. 522,* Geneva; World Health Organization, 1973.
69. H. Yoshimura, T. Inoue, T. Yamada, and K. Shiraki, *World Rev. Nutr. Diet.*, **35,** 1 (1980).

70. C. Meredith, D. M. Bier, N. M. Meguid, D. E. Matthews, Z. Wen, and V. R. Young, "Whole Body Amino Acid Turnover with ^{13}C Tracers: A New Approach for Estimation of Human Amino Acid Requirements," in R. I. C. Wesdorp and P. B. Soeters, Eds., *Clinical Nutrition '81,* Churchill Livingston, London, pp. 42–59.
71. C. F. Consolazio, H. L. Johnson, R. A. Nelson, J. G. Dramise, and J. H. Skala, *Am. J. Clin. Nutr.,* **28,** 29 (1975).
72. N. L. Marable, J. F. Hickson, Jr., M. K. Korslund, W. G. Herbert, R. F. Desjardins, and F. W. Thye, *Nutr. Repts. Intl.,* **19,** 795 (1979).
73. I. Celejowa and M. Homa, *Nutr. Metab.,* **12,** 259 (1970).
74. P. J. Rasch, J. W. Hamby, and H. J. Burns, *Med. Sci. Sports,* **1,** 195 (1969).
75. P. J. Rasch, and W. R. Piersan, *Am. J. Clin. Nutr.,* **11,** 530 (1962).
76. D. W. Barnett and R. K. Conlee, *Am. J. Clin. Nutr.,* **40,** 586 (1984).

3

Prescribing an Exercise Program

BERNARD GUTIN, Ph.D.

Teachers College, Columbia University, New York, New York

Exercise prescription should be effective and safe. That is, the exercise must be sufficiently stimulating to the physiological symptoms involved to cause an adaptation, but not so strenuous as to overwhelm or damage the body in the process.

It is generally agreed that people with any symptoms of heart disease, or major risk factors for cardiac disease, as well as any other medical problems that might require modification of the exercise prescription, should have a complete medical examination and stress test prior to a major alteration in their exercise habits. Although there are questions concerning the value of a stress test for diagnosis of disease in asymptomatic people (1), it is always useful to perform a functional fitness evaluation to provide a baseline against which progress may be measured and to serve as the foundation for the exercise prescription. Such a test should, at a minimum, measure heart rate response to exercise at a submaximal workrate and ideally would involve a multistage maximal test, with measurement of the ECG, blood pressure, rating of perceived exertion (RPE), oxygen consumption, and ventilatory breakpoint (VB, sometimes called anaerobic threshold). Measures of anaerobic fitness, body composition, and flexibility should also be included.

In prescribing exercise, we must consider first which components of fitness we would like to influence (Figure 3-1). There is no one test that can measure, or one type of exercise that will develop, all aspects of fitness. Emphasis is usually placed on aerobic fitness and body composition because of their importance in cardiovascular health and because the same type of exercise is valuable both for development of aerobic fitness and for consumption of a large number of calories. But a complete exercise program for adults should attend to strength and flexibility of the trunk and hip areas to help prevent back problems (2), and I believe that a few minutes of complete relaxation should be part of a complete exercise session. For young people interested in fitness for sports performance, anaerobic fitness, especially muscular power, is extremely important.

Fitness cannot be developed by some magical, painless technique that requires no work. On the other hand, it is not necessary to drive oneself to exhaustion every workout to achieve good results; some stimulation is necessary, but more is not necessarily better.

Figure 3-2 illustrates the general theory of fitness development. The individual imposes an overload on the system by doing more exercise than usual, eventually reaching a point of mild or severe fatigue. Then he allows a period of recovery to ensue,

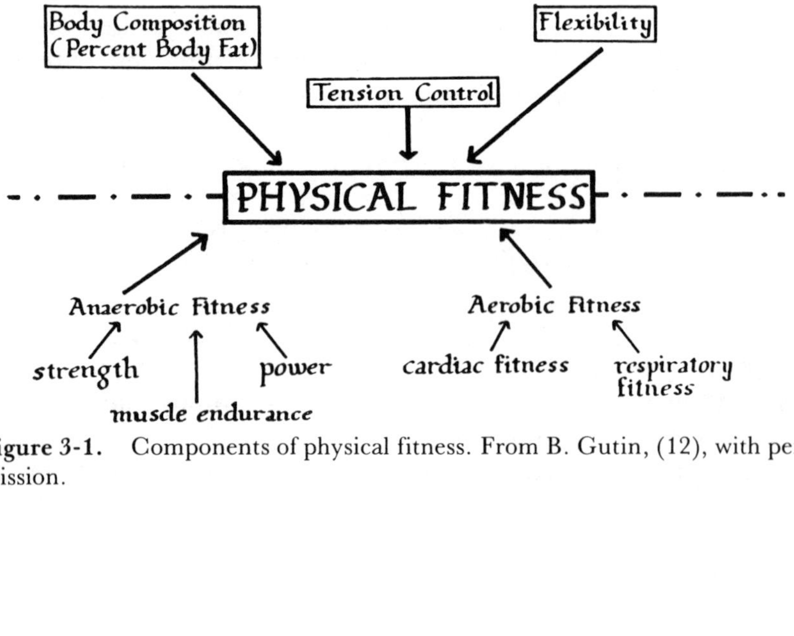

Figure 3-1. Components of physical fitness. From B. Gutin, (12), with permission.

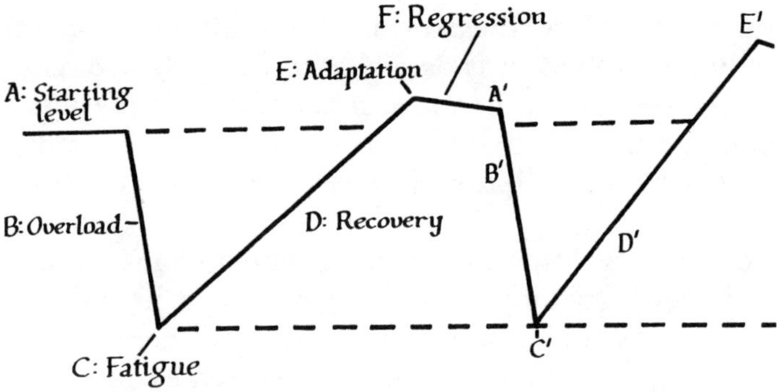

Figure 3-2. Theory of fitness development.

during which the systems stimulated respond to the stimulation by adapting up to a level of function that is greater than the starting level. Then the individual exercises again before too much regression takes place and the cycle is repeated. If he does this frequently enough, his work capacity will increase and he will have developed a "training effect." This general theory applies most clearly to anaerobic and aerobic fitness. For example, a given muscle may be stimulated to work at a submaximal workrate for 90 minutes, during which time the glycogen in the muscle will be depleted to relatively low levels. If a sufficient recovery period of 24–48 hours ensues, during which adequate carbohydrate is ingested, the glycogen level in the depleted muscles will rebound to a level higher than the one that existed before the workout (3). But rather than looking for illustrations of this theory in a particular system, it is better to think of it as applying to fitness development in general. Some corollaries to this theory are: (1) the overload must be of sufficient intensity and duration to be stimulating; (2) the recovery period must be long enough to allow adaptation to take place—for people just starting an exercise program it is often sensible to allow 48 hours or so, depending on how much of an overload was imposed; and (3) the workouts must be done frequently enough to assure that the adaptation gained from the last workout is not simply lost between sessions; that is, exercising only on weekends is of questionable fitness value.

Let us consider how these principles apply to aerobic fitness. As already mentioned, it is desirable to prescribe exercise based on a multistage test up to maximal capacity. If the test should be stopped short of maximal because of certain symptoms or signs, then the prescription is based on this "clinical maximum."

Figure 3-3 shows that as workrate increases in regular increments, oxygen consumption (VO_2) increases linearly up to a maximal level (VO_{2max}), after which further increases in workrate are not accompanied by further increases in VO_2. After training, submaximal VO_2 is usually unchanged, (i.e., the person does not become more mechanically efficient in well-learned tasks such as walking, running, or cycling), whereas VO_{2max} is usually increased.

Figure 3-4 shows that heart rate usually responds linearly to increments in workrate (or VO_2). After training, the resting and submaximal heart rates are reduced, while maximal heart rate changes very little. The beauty of using heart rate in exercise prescription is that the heart rate response is reduced as the individual becomes trained, so that he must work at a progressively higher workrate to reach the same heart rate.

A heart rate target zone of 60–90% of maximal heart rate (equivalent to approximately 50–85% of VO_{2max}) has been found

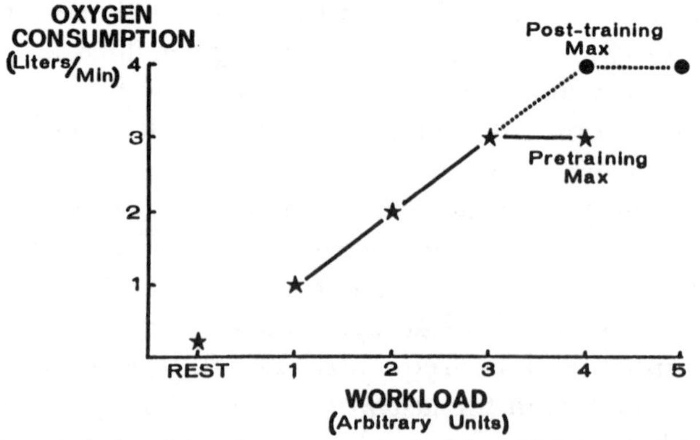

Figure 3-3. Relationship of oxygen consumption (VO_2) to workrate before and after training.

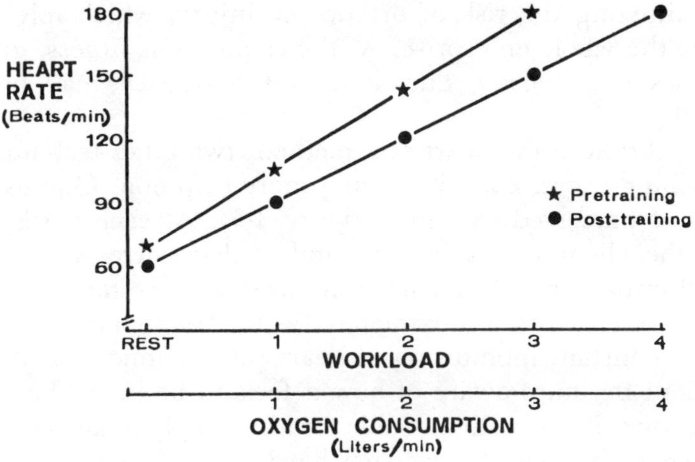

Figure 3-4. Relationship of heart rate to workrate and VO_2 before and after training. From B. Gutin (12), with permission.

to be effective in eliciting an aerobic training effect. If the maximal heart rate is known from the multistage test, then it should be used in the calculations. If not, then a rough estimate may be made by subtracting the person's age in years from 220 (e.g., a 40 year old has an estimated maximal heart rate of 180 beats per minute), keeping in mind that the standard deviation of the age-predicted maximal heart rate is 10–15 bpm.

If large leg muscle activity (e.g., walking, jogging, cycling, swimming, dancing, racquet sports) is used to raise heart rate into the target zone and keep it there for 15–60 minutes, and if workouts are carried out two to five times per week, good training results will occur (1). There are relationships among intensity, duration, and frequency, such that a greater intensity suggests that the individual reduce the duration of each workout. And if the combination of intensity and duration for a given session is relatively high, then the frequency of sessions may need to be reduced.

The main principle is to err on the side of caution by prescribing workouts at the lower end of the target zone for 15–30 minutes at a frequency of two to three times per week. This prescription should avoid feelings of fatigue after the workout as well as minimizing the risk of orthopedic injury, which might terminate the whole enterprise. As the client gains fitness, gradual increases in intensity, duration, and frequency may be prescribed.

In addition to the heart rate method, two other techniques of prescribing exercise are becoming more common. One uses the rating of perceived exertion (Figure 3-5). At each work increment the client indicates the number that corresponds to his overall impression of how hard the work is. The target zone for exercise intensity is approximately 12–16. For apparently healthy people, constant monitoring of heart rate is unnecessary. Once the client becomes aware of how it feels to be in the heart rate target zone, it is usually possible for him simply to keep the work somewhere between "somewhat hard" and "very hard" without stopping to measure his heart rate.

The target zone concept is simply empirical in nature, but a question that may be raised concerns what physiological events actually define this zone. One candidate for the lower end of the zone is the ventilatory breakpoint (VB) (also called the anaerobic threshold (AT) or lactate threshold—the correct terminology is

6	
7	**Very, very light**
8	
9	**Very light**
10	
11	**Fairly light**
12	
13	**Somewhat hard**
14	
15	**Hard**
16	
17	**Very hard**
18	
19	**Very, very hard**
20	

Figure 3-5. Rating of perceived exertion scale. From Gunnar Borg and Bruce J. Noble, "Perceived Exertion," in J. Wilmore, Ed. *Exercise and Sports Sciences Reviews, Vol. 2,* New York, Academic, 1974, with permission.

not yet settled). Figure 3-6 shows a model of some physiological responses to incremental work. As workrate increases, VO_2, ventilation (V_E), and expired CO_2 (VCO_2) increase linearly up to the VB (or AT), after which VO_2 continues to increase linearly while V_E and VCO_2 depart from linearity. It is at this point that plasma lactate values also begin to increase markedly. As workrate continues to rise, a point is reached at which V_E begins to increase out of proportion to increases in VCO_2. Apparently the body is responding with a respiratory alkalosis to compensate partially for the metabolic acidosis accompanying the rapid lactate accumulation, so that this point is called the respiratory compensation threshold (RCT). This may be the physiological

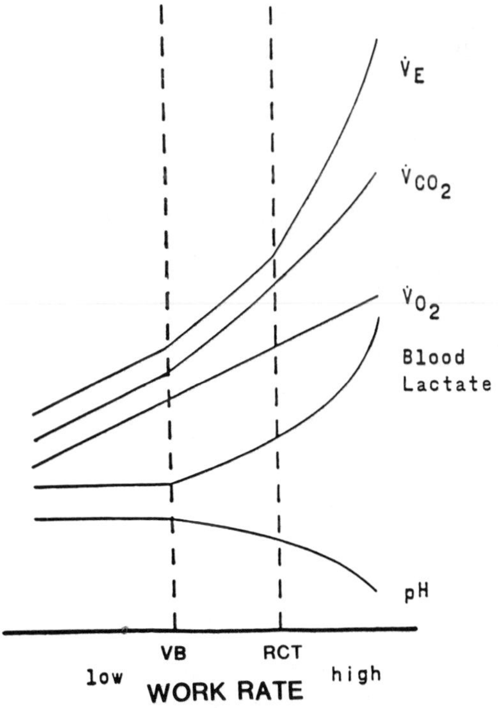

Figure 3-6. Physiological events associated with the anaerobic and respiratory compensation thresholds. Adapted from K. Wasserman, *New Eng. J. Med.*, **298,** 780 (1978), with permission.

upper limit for the target zone. Using physiologically determined indices of the upper and lower limits of the target zone should provide greater precision than may be gained from use of a given percent of VO_{2max}, which is only an indirect index of events transpiring at a submaximal level. Even though the 50–85% of VO_{2max} target zone corresponds on the average with the range between the VB and the RCT, individuals with the same VO_{2max} may have different VBs and RCTs, implying that their target zones should be different.

One implication of this concept is that if people are to pick a running speed at which they can continue for a long run, it will correspond to the treadmill speed at which these submaximal indices appear. Figure 3-7 shows that the critical running pace (CRP) adopted by men and women in a 3.2 km all-out run was higher, and not very closely correlated with (r = .69), the treadmill speed at which the VB (or AT) occurred. However, Figure

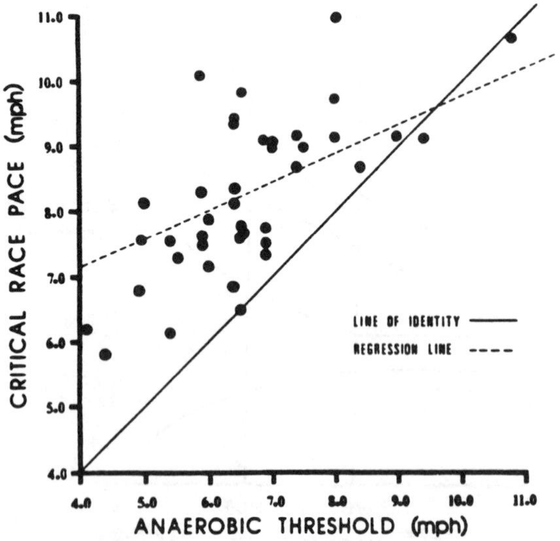

Figure 3-7. Critical race pace adopted in the middle 2.4 km of a 3.2 km all-out run in relation to the treadmill speed at which the anaerobic threshold (ventilatory breakpoint) was measured during an incremental test (r = .69). From C. Norton (4).

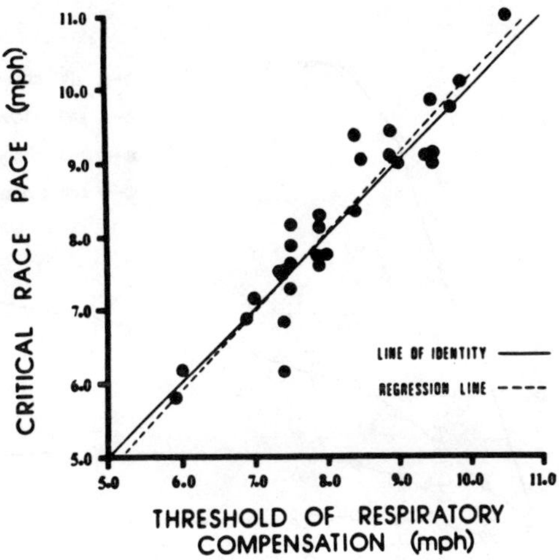

Figure 3-8. Critical race pace in relation to the treadmill speed corresponding to the threshold of respiratory compensation (r = .94). From C. Norton (4).

3-8 shows that the CRP was virtually identical to, and highly correlated with (r = .94), the treadmill speed at which the RCT appeared (4). More recently, it was shown (5) that for a longer distance, such as a marathon, people will select a speed very close to the VB (or AT).

We wanted to see what the pattern of lactate accumulation was in constant-load work carried out just below and just above the VB and RCT. Figure 3-9 shows that in work just above the VB (AT), plasma lactate reached a plateau at which lactate appearance and removal were in approximate equilibrium (6). At workrates just below the RCT, plasma lactate continued to increase gradually for 30 minutes, whereas at workrates just above the RCT it increased rapidly and no subject could complete the 30 minute workout. The mean was about 12 minutes.

Table 3-1 shows that even though plasma lactate and some other physiological measures plateaued, the RPE increased steadily throughout the workbout (7), perhaps because of other physiological changes taking place as the work continued (e.g., muscle glycogen depletion or increased temperature). Thus

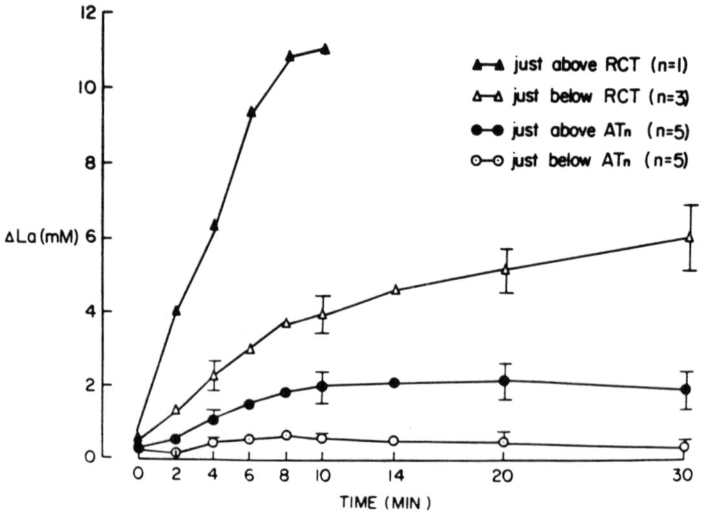

Figure 3-9. Delta Lactate response to constant load work just below and above the anaerobic threshold (ventilatory breakpoint) and the respiratory compensation threshold (RCT). From J. Simon and coworkers (6) with permission.

within this range RPE is a function of both intensity and duration of exercise.

We conducted a training study to see if good results might be obtained when the exercise was prescribed using the VB rather

Table 3-1. Physiological Values at the 10th, 20th, and 30th Minute of Work Just Above the Ventilatory Breakpoint (Anaerobic Threshold)[a]

Minute:	10	20	30
Rating of perceived exertion	13.0	14.2[b]	15.4[c]
Lactate (mmol/l)	3.2	3.4	3.2
Heart rate (bpm)	135	141	141
Ventilation (l/min)	53.8	55.1	56.6
Percent VO_{2max}	61.9	64.4[b]	65.3[b]

[a]From J. Simon, et al. (7) with permission.
[b]Significantly different from 10 minute value ($p < .05$).
[c]Significantly different from the 10 and 20 minute values ($p < .05$).

than percent of VO_{2max} (8). Table 3-2 shows that improvements in VO_{2max}, VB, and submaximal heart rates were very similar with the two methods of prescription. The RPEs after each workout were very similar under the two conditions even though the training heart rates for the 85% VO_{2max} method were approximately 9 bpm higher (167 versus 158 bpm). Since total distance covered each session was held constant, the people using the percent VO_{2max} method were finished sooner.

Even if you are unable to measure VB to prescribe exercise, it is important to realize that work at a given percent of VO_{2max} or maximal heart rate may be more or less taxing for a given individual depending on his submaximal fitness (i.e., VB or RCT), and should be used as a general guideline rather than a rigid prescription. Considering the ventilatory aspects of VB and RCT leads me to suggest a talk-sing concept for the target zone. If you cannot talk fairly easily, then you may be too close to your

Table 3-2. Changes in Physiologic Response to Exercise following 8 Weeks of Training Three Times per Week at 85% of VO_{2max} or Just Below Ventilatory Breakpoint (VB)[a]

		85% VO_{2max} ($n = 8$)	Ventilatory Breakpoint ($n = 6$)	Control ($n = 5$)
VO_{2max} (ml/kg/min)	pre	35.4	31.8	35.8
	post	39.2	35.6	35.4
	difference	3.8[b]	3.8	−0.4
VO_2 at VB (ml/kg/min)	pre	20.4	21.2	20.9
	post	24.3	23.4	20.8
	difference	3.9[b]	2.2	−0.1
HR at 3.5 mph, 6% grade (bpm)	pre	152	167	144
	post	141	148	145
	difference	−11[b]	−19*	1

[a]From B. Brehm (8). Subjects were 19 women with mean age of 27 years.
[b]$p < .05$ for pre-post difference.

RCT, whereas if your breathing is so easy that you can sing without difficulty you may be below the VB. So one way to estimate your target zone is to stay in the range where singing is difficult but talking is possible.

A recent issue in exercise prescription concerns the effect of assigning some work to the arms (e.g., carrying hand weights while jogging or walking). Figure 3-10 shows the VO_2 over 60 minutes of work just above the leg VB in which 0, 10, or 25% of the work was done with the arms (9). It is clear that VO_2 was higher in proportion to the amount of work done by the arms. Figures 3-11 and 3-12 show that cardiac output and heart rate were higher for the 25/75 condition but not for the 10/90 condition. Since blood pressures were lower when some of the work was assigned to the arms (Figure 3-13), the heart rate–systolic blood pressure product (Figure 3-14) was similar for all conditions. Furthermore, in the incremental tests done before these

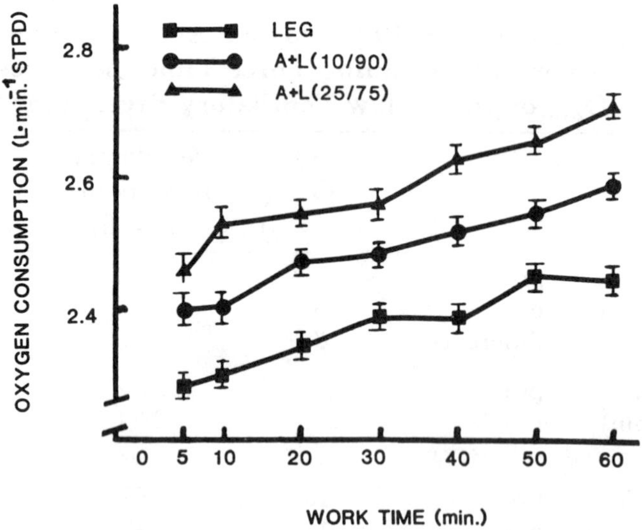

Figure 3-10. Oxygen consumption during constant load work at an intensity just above the leg ventilatory breakpoint when 0, 10, or 25% of the work was done by the arms (means ± SE). VO_2 increased significantly ($p < .05$) in all modes. The 25/75 mode was reliably higher than legs alone and the 10/90 mode was not reliably different from either. From K. Ang (9).

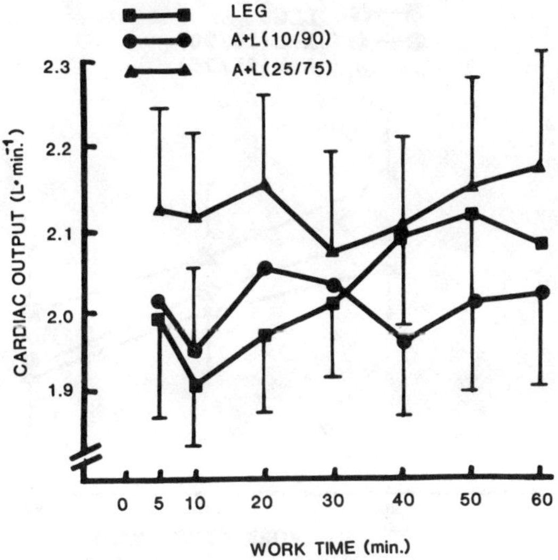

Figure 3-11. Cardiac output in combined arm and leg work. Values for the 25/75 mode were reliably higher ($p < .05$) than those of the other two modes, summed over time. From K. Ang (9).

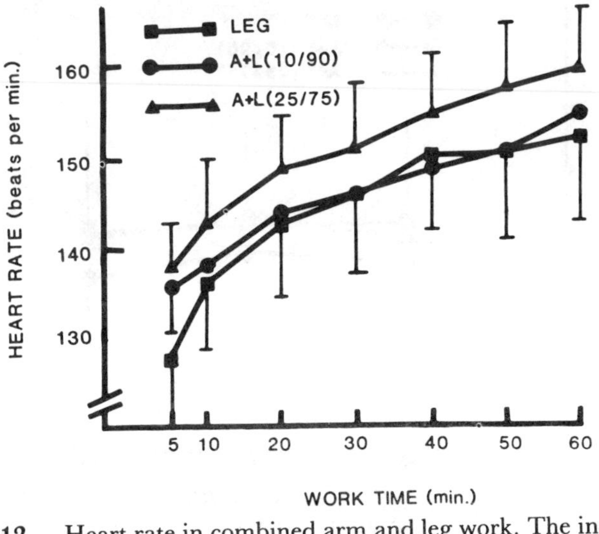

Figure 3-12. Heart rate in combined arm and leg work. The increases over time were significant ($p < .05$) but the differences among modes were not. From K. Ang (9).

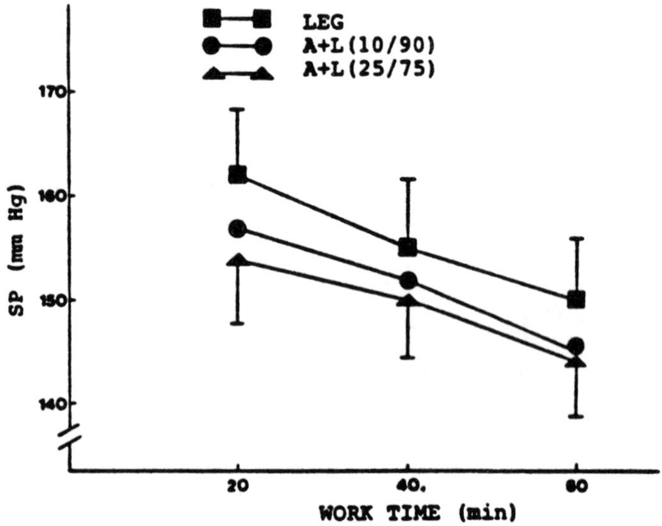

Figure 3-13. Systolic blood pressure in arm and leg work. The reduction over time was significant ($p < .05$), and the value of the leg mode summed over time was significantly greater than that of the 25/75 mode. From K. Ang (9).

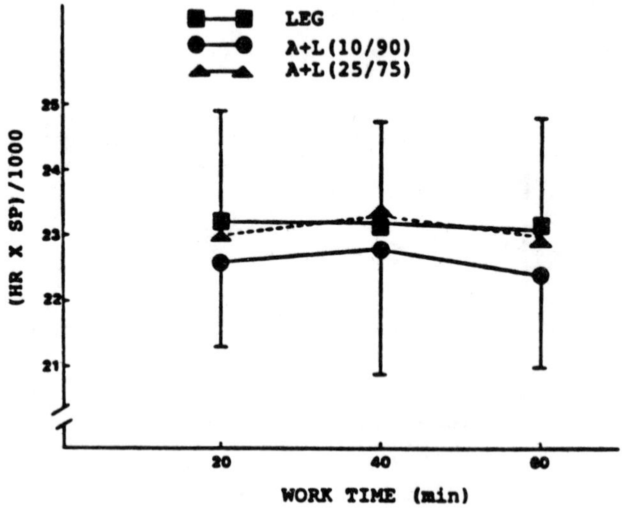

Figure 3-14. Heart rate–systolic blood pressure product in arm and leg work. None of the differences between modes or time periods was significant. From K. Ang (9).

prolonged work experiments the VB was significantly higher when 10% of the work was done by the arms. So as expected, the RPE during the prolonged work was somewhat lower when some of the work was done with the arms (Figure 3-15).

Thus it seems that assigning some of the work to the arms (i.e., spreading the work over a greater muscle mass) allows a greater metabolic load to be maintained with no greater cardiovascular or perceptual strain, conditions that seem desirable in exercise prescribed for aerobic fitness and weight control.

Should one warm up before taking part in an aerobic workout capped off by an all-out effort for the last few minutes? Figure 3-16 shows what happened when men warmed up for 20 minutes at various percentages of VO_{2max}, exercised for 10 minutes at 75% VO_{2max}, and then held out as long as possible while the treadmill speed was increased (10). Performance *declined* as the prior exercise increased in intensity. Thus aerobic activity seems to constitute its own warmup and doing prior exercise may actually deplete some resources unnecessarily. On the other hand,

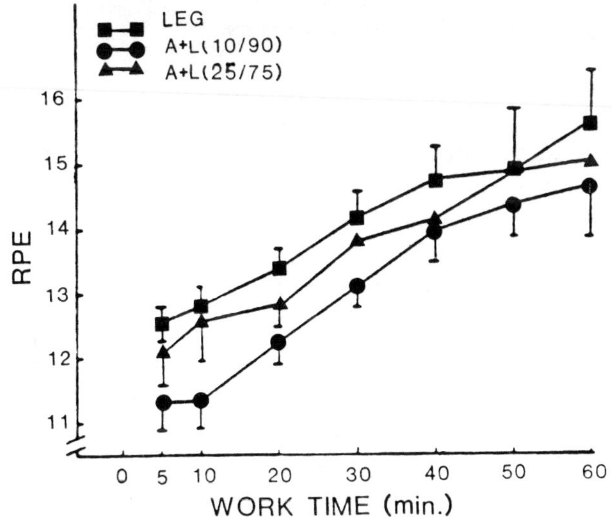

Figure 3-15. Rating of perceived exertion in arm and leg work. The increases over time periods were reliable ($p < .05$) but none of the differences among modes was. From K. Ang (9).

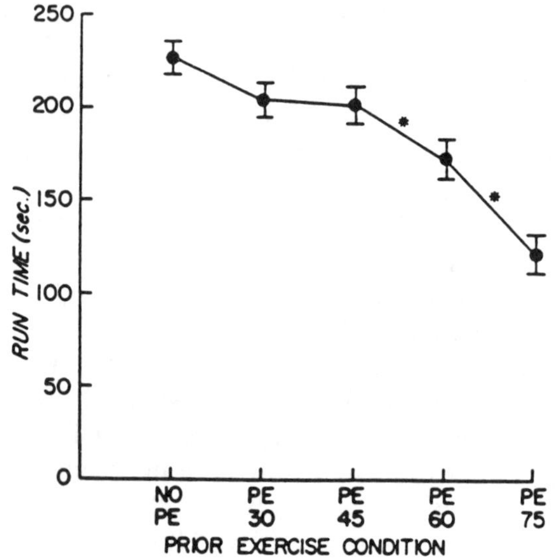

Figure 3-16. Run time following prior exercise at varying percentages of maximal oxygen consumption. The subjects walked for 20 minutes at the intensities shown, rested one minute, walked for 10 more minutes at 75% and then continued as long as possible while the treadmill speed was increased each subsequent minute. The asterisks indicate significant differences between means. From B. Gutin and coworkers (10) with permission.

if the exercise bout is to be at a very high intensity (i.e., anaerobic), then some mild prior exercise seems wise (11), especially if the ambient temperature is low.

If the ambient temperature is high, especially if accompanied by high relative humidity, it is important to maintain fluid balance by drinking often. Wearing a plastic suit to promote sweating and short term weight loss may be dangerous if it interferes with evaporation and leads to hyperthermia. Ironically, it is likely that the resulting limitations on how much work the person can do will reduce the total number of calories he can use up and actually be counterproductive for true weight loss.

In light of this discussion, what are the ingredients of a good exercise prescription? First, the exercise should engage a large muscle mass, as in walking, jogging, dancing, cycling, and swimming. Adding arm work, as in cross-country skiing, racquet sports, and hand weights, is sensible as a way of increasing the total load and conditioning more than one area of the body.

Second, impose a sufficent overload on the body in each session to call forth adaptive responses. The intensity should be in the target zone as defined by approximately 50–85% of VO_{2max}, 60–90% of maximal heart rate, an RPE of 12–16, or the "can talk-can't sing" ventilatory zone. The work should be "pleasurably tiring." If it is just pleasurable, you are probably not working hard enough. If it is just tiring, then you may be working too hard. Durations of 15–30 minutes early in training and up to 60 minutes as training progresses are desirable. Within the target zone, lower intensities can be balanced by greater durations and the training effect will be similar. Similarly, interval and continuous training will give similar results if the total work done is similar.

Third, carry out the exercise several times per week. Allowing a day off between sessions is sensible to minimize orthopedic problems, but as the client increases his capacity, he may be able to exercise every day. This is especially true if a variety of exercise modalities is used so that exactly the same muscles are not stressed each session. From the point of view of weight control, maximizing the total energy expenditure seems desirable (12).

Fourth, a complete session should attend to strength and flexibility by including calisthenics or weight lifting and static stretching for various parts of the body. I favor doing these after the aerobic phase of the session and I suggest ending with a few minutes of complete relaxation, lying on a relatively soft surface. It is easy to feel wonderfully relaxed after a good workout, and this type of reinforcement is likely to encourage the client to adopt on a permanent basis a high energy lifestyle.

REFERENCES

1. M. Pollock, J. Wilmore, and S. Fox, *Exercise in Health and Disease,* Saunders, Philadephia, 1984.
2. A. Melleby, *The Y's Way to a Healthy Back,* New Century, Piscataway, 1982.
3. E. Hultman, *Circulation Res.,* Suppl. 7, Vol. XX and XXI (March, 1967).

4. Cheryl Norton, Factors Affecting Circulorespiratory Endurance Performance, in Men and Women, Doctoral dissertation, Teachers College, Columbia University, 1980.
5. E. Rhodes and D. McKenzie, *The Physician & Sportsmedicine,* **12,** 95 (1984).
6. J. Simon, J. Young, B. Gutin, D. Blood, and R. Case, *J. Appl. Physiol.,* **54,** 13 (1983).
7. J. Simon, B. Gutin, J. Young, D. Blood, and R. Case, *Med. & Sci. in Sports and Exercise,* **16,** 140 (1984).
8. Barbara Brehm, "Choosing the Most Effective Exercise Intensity for Women's Physical Conditioning Program, M.A. project, Teachers College, Columbia University, 1979.
9. K. Ang, "Cardiorespiratory Response to Combined Arm and Leg Work," Doctoral dissertation, Teachers College, Columbia University, 1983.
10. B. Gutin, J. Wilkerson, S. Horvath, and R. Rochelle, *Intl. J. Sports Med.,* **2,** 87 (1981).
11. B. D. Franks, "Physical Warm-up," in M. Williams, Ed., *Ergogenic Aids in Sport,* Human Kinetics, Champaign, 1983.
12. B. Gutin, *The High Energy Factor,* Random House, New York, 1983.

4

Exercise, Diet, and Thermogenesis

JOHN S. GARROW, M.D.

Medical Research Council, Clinical Research Centre, Harrow, England

TWO PIONEERS IN HUMAN NUTRITION

I believe the greatest change that has taken place in research in human nutrition in the last few years has been the increased interest in the regulation of energy expenditure. Only 5 years ago the following passage appeared in a well-known British textbook of nutrition, concerning the etiology of obesity:

If a healthy man or woman eats only an extra slice of bread (20g) at breakfast, this provides a surplus of 200 kJ or 48 kcal of energy, which is stored as triglyceride. If he continues with this daily habit, after 10 years the store has grown by 20 kg and he has become very obese. Alternatively, if he takes his car to work instead of walking 10 minutes each way and does not reduce his food intake, the same surplus of energy has to be stored (1).

If we check on the arithmetic of this calculation we find that

$$48 \text{ kcal} \times 365 \text{ days} \times 10 \text{ years} = 175{,}200 \text{ kcal},$$

which is indeed roughly the energy value in 20 kg triglyceride, so the assumption implicit in the passage quoted above is that the intake of extra food has no effect on energy expenditure.

That assumption is no longer tenable in the light of recent work on the regulation of energy expenditure. I am particularly pleased and honored to dedicate this chapter to Dr. Hsien Wu, whose work in laying the foundations of modern nutritional biochemistry opened the way to a more rational investigation of human nutrition.

The work of Dr Wu, and the techniques that he established, were immediately adopted and used throughout the world. It is ironical that the understanding of thermogenesis in man that I shall describe is based on the work of a contemporary of Dr Wu, working just 100 miles to the northeast in Middletown, Connecticut. In 1919, when Hsein Wu completed his Ph.D. thesis entitled "A system of blood analysis," F. G. Benedict and his colleagues published their important work "Human vitality and efficiency under prolonged restricted diet" (2). This was the first great experimental study of human undernutrition, and the first to show conclusively that energy expenditure decreases in response to decreased energy intake. The topic of thermogenesis concerns the opposite adaptation: an increased expenditure in response to (among other things) increased energy intake. The techniques involved in this research were developed by Atwater and Benedict (3), but human nutritionists ceased to use them, because they are rather tedious, although animal nutritionists continued to use direct calorimetry. With the development of physical gas analyzers, and microprocessor control of direct calorimeters, it is once more possible without much difficulty to apply the techniques of both indirect and direct calorimetry to the problems of human nutrition.

DEFINITION OF THERMOGENESIS

Literally, thermogenesis means heat production, but in every metabolic reaction the energy involved is eventually degraded to heat, so the literal use of the word is too wide to be useful. It is now usual to use the term thermogenesis to describe the *increase* in metabolic rate that occurs in response to some stimulus such as exercise, food, or exposure to cold. If the thermogenic response is large, causing an increase many times the baseline level, some uncertainty about the baseline value does not matter very much. However, except in the case of exercise and exposure to severe cold, most thermogenic responses in man cause an increase of only a small fraction of the baseline metabolic rate, so in these circumstances we need to examine closely the precision of the baseline measurement.

Increase above what?

The statement that a given stimulus "causes an increase in metabolic rate of x%" or "of y kcal" implies that the metabolic rate without the stimulus is known, but often this is not so. It is not uncommon to see a report of the metabolic rate measured after a test stimulus based on the assumption that, had the stimulus not been applied, the metabolic rate would have remained exactly at the level that had been observed before the stimulus was given. This may be so, but it has to be established by suitable control measurements under identical conditions, but without the stimulus.

There are two reasons for caution in assuming constancy of the baseline metabolic rate. First, any measurement over several hours in a ventilated hood apparatus, or even more so with a facemask or mouthpiece, is tedious or even uncomfortable for the subject, so any increase in metabolic rate may in part indicate restiveness with the experimental procedure rather than a true thermogenic response to the stimulus. Second, it is common to conduct experiments on thermogenesis starting in the early morning, and often continuing into the afternoon. This is a period in which the circadian rhythm of energy metabolism is increasing, so if a constant baseline is assumed the thermogenic effect will be overestimated. Both these sources of error will be avoided if the appropriate control measurement is made. This advice to students of human thermogenesis may be enshrined thus:

RULE 1. DO NOT ASSUME THE BASELINE IS CONSTANT.
The cause of the circadian rhythm in energy metabolism is not clear. It persists even when people are maintained under constant conditions, so it is not simply a daily response to lighting conditions or patterns of social activity. It has even been shown in birds which are normally active in the daytime that the increase in metabolic activity will occur around midday for many days under totally constant conditions, while night-active birds such as the owl will continue to have peak metabolic activity at night (4).

DOES THERMOGENESIS MATTER?

Thermoregulatory thermogenesis is of vital importance to small mammals. To maintain physiological body temperature in a cold environment they must be able to generate heat to keep pace with inevitable heat losses by conduction, convection, radiation, and evaporation. For a given temperature gradient between the body and the environment heat loss by radiation is proportional to surface area, and to a lesser extent this is true also of convection and conduction. A typical mouse weighing 100 g may have a surface area of about 0.1 mz, so the surface area/weight ratio is about 1 m^2/kg. A large mammal, like man, typically has a body weight of 70 kg and a surface area of 1.73 m^2, so the surface area/weight ratio is 0.025 m^2/kg, or about 40 times less than that of a mouse. Perhaps another dictum for students of thermogenesis could be stated thus:

RULE 2. DO NOT EXTRAPOLATE FROM MOUSE TO MAN
Much of the recent interest in thermogenesis in small laboratory rodents arises from the possibility that they may provide a clue to the etiology of human obesity (5). It is well established that several strains of genetically obese mice and rats have a reduced capacity for cold-induced thermogenesis (6–8) but whether this defect, and specifically a defect in brown adipose tissue, can be generalized to a defect in diet-induced thermogenesis is a matter of debate (9, 10). My own views on this controversy are recorded

elsewhere (11); for the moment I will concentrate on evidence that bears directly on man, in accordance with the precepts stated in Rule 2 above.

RESTING METABOLISM IN LEAN AND OBESE HUMAN SUBJECTS

So far as I know, every study of the thermogenic response of lean and obese subjects has agreed on at least one point: the mean baseline energy expenditure of the obese group was higher than the mean of the lean group (12–18). This is a remarkable degree of unanimity among so many different laboratories. We have found no evidence that obese people who had characteristics which might indicate a genetic disposition to obesity, such as obesity of childhood onset, or a family history of obesity, have any lower resting metabolic rate than obese people without these characteristics (19). This is important, because it shows that if there is a form of human obesity which is characterized by low energy expenditure then this variant must be rare (and hence not detected in the groups studied so far), or else the economy in energy expenditure must be effected in aspects other than resting energy expenditure—in other words in reduced thermogenesis.

A possible alternative hypothesis is that human obesity is initially associated with a decreased resting metabolic rate, but with increasing obesity this effect is masked by the increase in both fat and nonfat tissues which is characteristic of human (but not rodent) obesity (20). This hypothesis is hard to test, since it involves investigating individuals who are going to become obese, but who are not obese yet, and such subjects are obviously difficult to identify and study. There are two points of indirect evidence against the idea that obese subjects would have a low resting metabolic rate if they were not obese. First, in a regression analysis of resting metabolic rate on body composition in 140 women, the best fit equation contained a term for body weight and a term for lean body mass, both of which contributed significantly to the regression, and both of which had a positive sign

(21). In other words, for women of similar lean body mass the heavier women had the higher metabolic rate. If obesity was initially associated with a low metabolic rate, which was raised only by the addition of extra fat and nonfat tissue, we would have expected that the term for weight in the regression equation would have had a negative sign. The other piece of evidence which points against an underlying hypometabolic state in obese people is the observation that after massive weight loss the resting metabolic rate of formerly obese women is not lower than that of women of similar age and body composition who had never been very obese (21).

EXERCISE-INDUCED THERMOGENESIS

Physical activity is by far the most potent thermogenic stimulus in man. Its nearest rival is exposure to severe cold: after 2 hours in an air temperature of 5°C the resting metabolic rate of lightly clad subjects roughly doubles (22), but a similar increase in metabolic rate could have been achieved by quite light physical activity, such as walking at 5 km/hour on level ground (23). Indeed the energy cost of strenuous physical activity may exceed the capacity of the heart and lungs to transport oxygen to the working muscles, so anaerobic pathways of metabolism are used and an oxygen debt is incurred.

Duration of Elevated Metabolism

Proponents of the thermogenic power of physical activity claim that a substantial portion of the energy cost of exercise occurs in the elevated metabolism after the exercise ceases. "Thus half an hour of squash may expend only 450 kcal. However the increase in metabolic rate over the ensuing two days could account for possibly another 550 kcal (approximately), making a total of 1000 kcal" (24). This calculation is unduly optimistic. First, it is unlikely that the average rate of energy expenditure while playing squash for 30 minutes would be 15 kcal/minute. This rate of metabolism might be reached for short periods during rallies, but not maintained throughout the entire game. The suggestion that another 550 kcal might be expended over the next 48 hours is more difficult to test; this implies an average increase in metabolic rate of 0.2 kcal/minute, which would be difficult to detect.

The results of an attempt to measure the duration of elevated metabolic rate after exercise are shown in Figure 4-1. In this study normal young women rode a bicycle ergometer at 50 revolutions per minute against a load of 1 kp for 20 minutes each hour for 4 consecutive hours. This workload was chosen as being within the capacity of reasonably fit women, but our subjects could not have worked at this load for a longer period, or with more repetitions. For the first 2.3 hours the subjects were fasting, then a meal supplying 800 kcal was eaten during a 20 minute period, and then another 2.3 hours was done. The subjects also performed control experiments over the same period, with the same dietary input, but without the exercise.

The average rate of energy expenditure for each resting and exercising period was measured by continuous indirect calorimetry (25), the vertical bars indicate 1 SEM. The lower part of the histogram with diagonal shading indicates the metabolic rate during the control, nonexercising studies. In the fasting state the metabolic rate is about 1 kcal/minute and quite constant; after the meal there is an increase of about 10–15%.

The energy expenditure during the exercising periods is indicated by the stippled bars; this is about 5 times the resting level. However immediately after the exercise stops the metabolic rate falls almost to the control level. The solid bands on the periods after exercise indicate the increase in metabolic rate post-exercise compared with the control measurements. There is an increase of about 0.2 kcal/minute for the 40 minutes immediately following the exercise, but this increment does not accumulate and become progressively bigger with successive exercise bouts.

A similar conclusion was reached in a study by 24 hour direct calorimetry of lean and obese women after moderate exercise: the energy cost over the 24 hours was no greater than that which would be expected from the energy expended during the exercise (18). It seems, therefore, that there is little or no prolongation

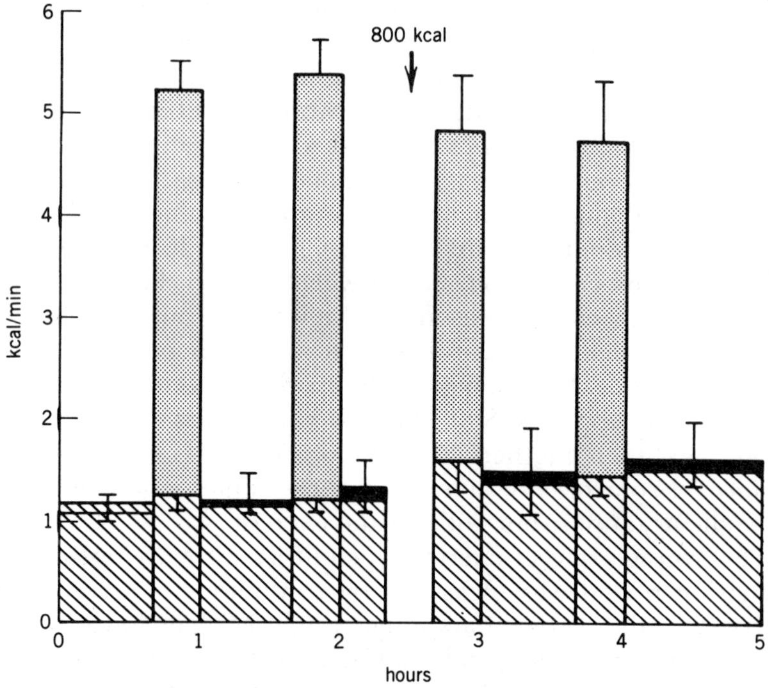

Figure 4-1. Energy expenditure in normal women at rest, before and after a meal (diagonally shaded area), and during periods of exercise (stippled area). Note that there is no potentiation of the thermogenic effect of exercise by the meal, and that the metabolic rate falls almost to control levels immediately after the exercise period is finished. (Unpublished data of P. Pacy, J. D. Webster, N. Barton, and J. S. Garrow.)

of the raised metabolic rate after moderate exercise, but there seem to be few well-controlled studies on the effect of strenuous exercise on subsequent metabolic rate.

The Effect of Exercise on 24 Hour Energy Expenditure

From their extensive review of the literature Passmore and Durnin (23) conclude that an average rate of work of 5 kcal/minute over an 8 hour working day is the maximum that can be performed for 6 days a week, week after week. They calculate that 8 hours of heavy work costs 2400 kcal, 8 hours in bed costs about 500 kcal, and the remaining 8 hours spent off work would typically cost about 1400 kcal, making a total of 4300 kcal, which agrees well with the upper limit of measured energy costs of very heavy industrial work.

Because more than half the daily energy expenditure occurs at work (2400 out of 4300 kcal) it has been suggested that physical activity can double daily energy expenditure. This is false arithmetic. Suppose the heavy manual worker had not done any heavy work, but had spent the day in his usual off-duty activities. His energy expenditure would have been 1400 kcal for that period instead of 2400 kcal. Thus the saving from not working is only 1000 kcal, not 2400 kcal, so the work costs less than a quarter of the total, not more than a half. An example of the effect of heavy manual work on energy expenditure comes from a study on coal miners working at the coalface with picks and shovels, compared with colleagues at the surface doing clerical jobs (26). The miners had an average expenditure of 3660 kcal/day, while the clerks averaged 2800 kcal/day.

Of course, highly trained athletes regularly achieve higher rates of energy expenditure than this during competition. A good marathon runner will maintain an oxygen uptake of about 4 liters/minute for 2 hours, which indicates an expenditure of about 2500 kcal during the race. Competitors in a 24 hour cross-country ski race may maintain an expenditure of 5 kcal/minute throughout the 24 hours, giving a total of 7000 kcal in a day, but they will not repeat this performance day after day.

DIET-INDUCED THERMOGENESIS IN LEAN AND OBESE SUBJECTS

It can be seen from Figure 4-1 that the magnitude of the thermogenic response to food is far smaller than that to exercise, so this response is technically more difficult to measure.

Thermogenesis Induced by a Single Meal

The original work on the thermogenic effect of food was done by Max Rubner on dogs. He noted that there was a greater increase in metabolic rate after a meal of meat than after an isoenergetic meal of sugar or lard (which will not surprise anyone who has fed a dog). The effect was called "specific dynamic action of protein," but in man the thermic effect of isoenergetic nonprotein meals is not very different (25). The time-course of the increase in metabolic rate above control level differs after carbohydrate, protein, or fat meals. After a glucose load metabolic rate rises to a peak at about 45 minutes, and is declining again by 2 hours after the meal. With a protein meal the peak response is about 1.5 to 2 hours after the meal, and metabolic rate does not return to control levels for several hours. With a fat meal (double cream) the increase in metabolic rate is small and gradual, with no clearly defined peak. Thus the measured thermogenic response depends on the duration of measurement: if metabolic rate is measured for 2 hours after the meal virtually the whole of the glucose response will be measured, but only part of the response to protein or fat (17).

The literature is contradictory about the relative magnitude of diet-induced thermogenesis in lean and obese subjects, partly for the technical reasons described above, and partly because some workers report the thermic effect of a meal as percent increase over resting metabolism in the subject, rather than as percent of the energy value of the meal. Since the obese subjects invariably have a higher resting metabolism, if the same absolute response to a meal is obtained in both lean and obese subjects for the same size of meal, this will appear as a smaller percent increase in metabolism in the obese group.

Even if the response is expressed as an absolute increase in metabolism, or as a proportion of the energy value in the meal, there is still no consensus about the thermogenic responsiveness of lean and obese subjects. We have failed to find any decrease in thermogenic response to carbohydrate, protein, or fat meals in obese subjects compared with our normal controls (17). When our results are compared with those from laboratories who report a decreased response in obese subjects the difference lies in the very low baseline metabolic rate of their lean "control" subjects. It may be, therefore, that there are some thin people who have a low resting metabolic rate which increases greatly after a meal, and compared with these the response of obese subjects is decreased. However, compared with these people the response of our normal controls is also decreased. At any rate, this decreased thermogenic response to food cannot in itself explain the obesity, since even after the meal the total energy output of the obese group is greater than that of the controls.

Thermogenesis Induced by Chronic Overfeeding

The most important study of experimental overfeeding of normal volunteers was that carried out by the Vermont group (27). The weight gained during the period of overfeeding was much less than would be expected if there had been no compensatory change in energy output, but unfortunately energy expenditure was not systematically studied in that experiment. Most subsequent studies in which normal volunteers were overfed by a substantial amount found an increase in resting metabolism (28), but the authors have differed in their interpretation of this finding. For example Norgan and Durnin (29) observed about a 10% increase in metabolic rate after 42 days of overfeeding, and attributed this to the metabolic activity of the weight that had been gained, while Dauncey (30) observed a similar increase in metabolic rate after only 1 day of overfeeding, when weight gain cannot have been the explanation.

A particularly interesting study is that of Webb and Annis (31) who overfed seven lean and five obese subjects by 1000 kcal/day for 30 days. They observed a similar increase both in body weight (2.5 kg and 2.2 kg) and in metabolic rate (7.3% and 7.5%) in lean and obese groups, respectively. This result does not support the often-expressed view that lean people are so constituted that they can eat unlimited amounts of food without weight gain, because they "burn it off," while obese people readily gain weight on any excess intake. Indeed the authors say that they recruited their lean subjects because they had always been lean, and the obese subjects had a history of gaining weight easily (31).

INTERACTION OF DIET AND EXERCISE IN CAUSING THERMOGENESIS

It has been suggested that the thermogenesis induced by food and exercise is more than additive, in other words, that thermogenesis induced by a meal has the effect of increasing the cost of subsequent exercise over the cost of the same exercise in the fasting state (32). No such additive effect can be seen in Figure 4-1; indeed the energy cost of the two exercise bouts after the meal is lower than that of similar exercise before the meal, but not significantly so.

Other experiments have also failed to confirm the effect described by Miller and Wise (32). In obese Pima Indians a period of overfeeding by 1000 kcal/day for 3 weeks increased resting metabolic rate but had no effect on the energy cost of bicycle ergometer work (33). Garby and Lammert (34) measured the energy cost of work on a bicycle ergometer in subjects whose dietary intake had been either 4 MJ or 18 MJ on the previous day, and failed to find any effect of the previous day's intake on the energy cost of the work. Dallosso and James (35) increased the intake of subjects 50% above maintenance requirements by increasing dietary fat, and did not find any change in the energy cost of work, measured by 24 hour calorimetry. In a variety of protocols, therefore, no interaction of diet and exercise has been found in causing an enhancement of the thermogenic response.

Thermoregulatory thermogenesis is of vital importance to small mammals, but man (in normal circumstances) has no requirement to generate heat to maintain body temperature. The heat generated as a by-product of normal metabolism is enough to compensate for normal heat losses.

In man, exercise is by far the most powerful thermogenic stimulus, which can increase metabolic rate 15 times above resting levels. However, other constraints limit the increase in habitual daily energy expenditure that can be achieved by exercise to 800-1000 kcal per day for normally physically fit people. There is no convincing evidence for an interaction between diet-induced and exercise-induced thermogenesis in man, or of a prolonged thermogenic effect of exercise after the activity ceases.

Diet-induced thermogenesis typically accounts for about 10% of the energy expenditure of subjects in energy balance. There is no convincing evidence that obese people have a reduced thermogenic response to food either as a single meal or as chronic overfeeding, but the average energy expenditure of a group of obese subjects (whether in the fed or fasted state) is consistently found to be higher than that of control groups of normal weight.

Recent advances in the study of thermogenesis have given us no reason to reject the views on the etiology of obesity which were expressed in conversation with Mr James Boswell by Dr Samuel Johnson, the well-known lexicographer (36). Talking of a man who had grown very fat, so as to be much incommoded by his corpulency, he said:

	"He eats too much, Sir."
BOSWELL:	"I don't know, Sir. You will see one man fat who eats moderately and another lean who eats a great deal."
JOHNSON:	"Nay, Sir, *whatever the quantity that a man eats* it is plain that if he is too fat he has eaten more than he should have done."

Note that the shrewd Dr Johnson has avoided the trap of saying that the obese person must have eaten more than a lean person does, and we also should avoid that statement, because it may not be true. However, as a summary of the cause of human obesity this statement by a nonmedical doctor, made over 200 years ago, can not be refuted by any insights gained by modern research.

REFERENCES

1. S. Davidson, R. Passmore, J. F. Brock, and A. S. Truswell, *Human Nutrition and Dietetics,* 7th ed., Churchill Livingstone, Edinburgh, 1979, p. 246.
2. F. G. Benedict, W. R. Miles, P. Roth, and M. Smith, *Human Vitality and Efficiency under Prolonged Restricted Diet,* Carnegie Institution Publication 280, Washington, 1919, p. 701.
3. W. O. Atwater and F. G. Benedict, *A Respiration-Calorimeter with Appliances for the Direct Determination of Oxygen,* Carnegie Institution Publication 42, Washington, 1905, p. 193.
4. J. Ashoff and H. Pohl, *Fed. Proc.,* **29,** 1541 (1970).
5. J. Himms-Hagen, *Can. Med. Assn. J.,* **121,** 1361 (1979).
6. T. R. A. Davis and J. Mayer, *Am. J. Physiol.,* **177,** 222 (1954).
7. M. L. Kaplan and G. A. Leveille, *Am. J. Physiol.,* **227,** 912 (1974).
8. P. L. Thurlby, P. Trayhurn, and W. P. T. James, *Proc. Nutr. Soc. (Lond.),* **35,** 133A (1976).
9. N. J. Rothwell and M. J. Stock, *Clin. Sci.,* **64,** 19 (1983).
10. G. R. Hervey and G. Tobin, *Clin. Sci.,* **64,** 7 (1983).
11. J. S. Garrow, *Brit. Med. J.,* **286,** 1684 (1983).
12. Ph. Pittet, Ph. Chappuis, K. Acheson, F. de Techtermann, and E. Jequier, *Brit. J. Nutr.,* **35,** 281 (1976).
13. M. L. Kaplan and G. A. Leveille, *Am. J. Clin. Nutr.,* **29,** 1108 (1976).
14. P. S. Shetty, R. T. Jung, W. P. T. James, M. A. Barrand, and B. A. Callingham, *Clin. Sci.,* **60,** 519 (1981).
15. J. B. Morgan, D. A. York, A. Wasilewska, and J. Portman, *Brit. J. Nutr.,* **47,** 21 (1982).
16. N. N. Sharief and I. Macdonald, *Am. J. Clin. Nutr.,* **35,** 267 (1982).
17. K. S. Nair, D. Halliday, and J. S. Garrow, *Clin. Sci.,* **65,** 307 (1983).
18. S. Blaza and J. S. Garrow, *Brit. J. Nutr.,* **49,** 171 (1983).
19. J. S. Garrow, S. E. Blaza, P. M. Warwick, and M. A. Ashwell, *Lancet,* **i,** 1103 (1980).
20. J. D. Webster, R. Hesp, and J. S. Garrow, *Hum. Nutr. Clin. Nutr.,* **38C,** 299 (1984).
21. C. Dore, R. Hesp, D. Wilkins, J. S. Garrow, *Hum. Nutr. Clin. Nutr.,* **36C,** 41 (1982).
22. C. H. Wyndham, C. G. Williams, and H. Loots, *J. Appl. Physiol.,* **24,** 282 (1968)
23. R. Passmore and J. V. G. A. Durnin, *Physiol. Rev.,* **35,** 801 (1955).
24. D. W. Allen and B. M. Quigley, *Med. J. Austr.,* **2,** 434 (1977).
25. J. S. Garrow and S. F. Hawes, *Brit. J. Nutr.,* **27,** 211 (1972).
26. R. C. Garry, R. Passmore, G. M. Warnock, and J. V. G. A. Durnin, *Studies on Expenditure of Energy and Consumption of Food by Miners and Clerks, Fife, Scotland,* M.R.C. Spec Rep. Ser. No. 289, H.M.S.O., London, 1955.

27. E. A. H. Sims, E. Danforth, Jr., E. S. Horton, G. A. Bray, J. A. Glennon, and L. B. Salans, *Rec. Prog. Hormone Res.*, **29**, 457 (1973).

28. J. S. Garrow, "Regulation of Energy Expenditure in Man," in G. Bray, Ed., *Recent Advances in Obesity Research,* Newman, London, 1978, pp. 200–210.

29. N. G. Norgan and J. V. G. A. Durnin, *Am. J. Clin. Nutr.*, **33**, 978 (1980).

30. M. J. Dauncey, *Brit. J. Nutr.*, **43**, 257 (1980).

31. P. Webb and J. F. Annis, *Hum. Nutr. Clin. Nutr.*, **37C**, 117 (1983).

32. D. S. Miller and A. Wise, *Lancet,* **i**, 1290 (1975).

33. E. Danforth, Jr., R. J. Daniels, H. L. Katzeff, E. Ravussin, and J. S. Garrow, *Clin. Res.*, **29**, 663A (1981).

34. L. Garby and O. Lammert, *Acta Physiol. Scand.*, **101**, 411 (1977).

35. H. M. Dallosso and W. P. T James, *Brit. J. Nutr.*, **52**, 65 (1984).

36. J. Boswell, *The Applause of the Jury, 1782–1785,* I. S. Lustig and F. A. Pottle, Eds., Heinemann, London, p. 118.

5

Nutritional Enhancement of Athletic Performance

JACK H. WILMORE, Ph.D.
and BEAU J. FREUND

University of Arizona, Tucson, Arizona

For centuries, athletes have searched for the perfect diet, one that will assure them of attaining their optimal peak performance during sports competition. As a result of an intense desire to be successful, most athletes become both experimenter and subject, attempting by trial and error to identify that one factor or combination of factors which will give them the winning edge. Consequently, athletic nutrition has evolved largely through tradition and self-experimentation, with relatively few well-controlled studies to guide the scientist, clinician, coach, trainer, and athlete. Since the early 1960s, increased research efforts have been directed towards better defining optimal athletic nutrition, including investigations of specific nutrients to determine their potential ergogenic or performance-enhancing attributes.

This chapter reviews the more recent work on nutrition as it relates to athletic performance. Most of this review will focus on the aerobic or cardiovascular endurance aspects of athletic performance since this represents the largest available body of knowledge. Discussion will center on the role of protein, fats, and carbohydrates, and vitamins and minerals, in the optimization of athletic performance.

PROTEIN, FATS, AND CARBOHYDRATES

There is agreement on the relative nutrient demands of the athlete concerning the percentage of energy to be derived from protein, fats, and carbohydrates (1–4). Proteins should constitute 10–15% of the total energy, or 1.0–1.5 grams of protein per kilogram of body weight (g/kg). Fats should be limited to 30–35% of the total energy, with saturated fats constituting less than 10% of the total. Carbohydrates would make up the balance. For athletes who have extraordinary energy demands, that is, who expend an additional 8.38 MJ (2000 kcal) to 16.76 MJ (4000 kcal) per day in practice or in competition, the relative contribution may change, with carbohydrates providing 70% or more of the total energy consumed. This recommendation comes from the work of Costill and his associates (5,6). They demonstrated that subjects who trained heavily and were maintained on a relatively low carbohydrate diet, that is, approximately 40% of total energy, had a steady decline in muscle glycogen levels with successive days of training. When these same subjects were fed a diet high in carbohydrate, that is, approximately 70% of total energy, but of equal energy content, muscle glycogen levels remained relatively stable. The importance of maintaining high muscle glycogen levels will be discussed later in this chapter.

In addition to the relative contribution of each of the nutrients, consideration must be given to the total calories consumed. Although this is highly variable dependent on the size, sex, and the sport of the athlete, values as high as 50.3 MJ (12,000 kcal) per day have been reported (7). Athletes in certain sports, such as wrestling, boxing, and horse racing, must monitor their weight carefully to meet established standards for competition. This has led to nutritional abuses, dehydration, and increased risk of heat stress and renal ischemia (8). In addition, there is increasing concern regarding the nutritional behaviors used to achieve excessive weight losses in athletes, and their potential association with eating disorders, such as anorexia nervosa and the bulimia-purging syndrome (9).

At the other extreme, it has been our personal observation (unpublished) that athletes in certain sports have difficulty in maintaining their desired weight, that is, they experience a gradual weight loss over the course of a season. These individuals appear to have difficulty consuming sufficient energy to maintain body weight. Swimmers and runners will frequently fall into this category. As an example, a male world-class swimmer 16 years of age and 65 kg of body weight may have a normal energy expenditure of 12.8 MJ (3070 kcal)/day (10). With 4 hours of swim training in the pool, and 1 hour of dry land drills, an additional 3.35 MJ (800 kcal)/hour would be spent, amounting to 16.75 MJ (4000 kcal) in 5 hours, or a total of 29.55 MJ (7070 kcal) in 24 hours. With such high rates of energy expenditure, the need for sleep increases, with 12 hours per night or more being quite common. With 12 hours of sleep, and 5 hours of exercise, the athlete is left with 7 hours in which to ingest over 29 MJ.

To determine total energy intake needs, it is first necessary to define the optimal body composition for that individual to determine if weight should remain the same, be reduced or increased. Wilmore (11) has recently reviewed the body composition literature for athletes of both sexes in a wide variety of sports. A summary of this review is presented in Table 5-1, which can be used as a guide in determining the optimal performance weight for the individual athlete. Once that weight has been established, the athlete's energy expenditure over 24 hours can be estimated and the energy intake adjusted accordingly.

PROTEIN NEEDS

Do the protein needs of the athlete differ from those of the average sedentary individual? Do protein requirements differ for athletes in different sports? For a number of years it was assumed that athletes should consume large quantities of protein, either through high protein foods, or through protein supplements. This assumption possibly evolved from early beliefs that the muscle consumed itself as fuel for its contractions, and that supplementation of protein was essential to prevent general muscle atrophy from chronic exercise. More recently, attention has focused on

Table 5-1. Body composition values in male and female athletes[a]

Athletic Group or Sport	Sex	Age (yr)	Height (cm)	Weight (kg)	Relative (Fat (%)	Reference
Baseball	male	20.8	182.7	83.3	14.2	(12)
	male	—	—	—	11.8	(13)
	male	27.4	183.1	88.0	12.6	Wilmore, unpublished
Basketball	female	19.1	169.1	62.6	20.8	(14)
	female	19.4	167.0	63.9	26.9	(15)
Centers	male	27.7	214.0	109.2	7.1	(16)
Forwards	male	25.3	200.6	96.9	9.0	(16)
Guards	male	25.2	188.0	83.6	10.6	(16)
Canoeing	male	23.7	182.0	79.6	12.4	(17)
Football	male	20.3	184.9	96.4	13.8	(12)
	male	—	—	—	13.9	(13)
Defensive backs	male	17-23	178.3	77.3	11.5	(18)
	male	24.5	182.5	84.8	9.6	(19)
Offensive backs	male	17-23	179.7	79.8	12.4	(18)
	male	24.7	183.8	90.7	9.4	(19)
Linebackers	male	17-23	180.1	87.2	13.4	(18)
	male	24.2	188.6	102.2	14.0	(19)
Offensive linemen	male	17-23	186.0	99.2	19.1	(18)
	male	24.7	193.0	112.6	15.6	(19)

Defensive linemen	male	17-23	186.6	97.8	18.5	(18)
	male	25.7	192.4	117.1	18.2	(19)
Quarterbacks, kickers	male	24.1	185.0	90.1	14.4	(19)
Gymnastics	male	20.3	178.5	69.2	4.6	(12)
	female	19.4	163.0	57.9	23.8	(15)
	female	20.0	158.5	51.5	15.5	(20)
	female	14.0	—	—	17.0	(21)
	female	23.0	—	—	11.0	(21)
	female	23.0	—	—	9.6	(22)
Ice hockey	male	26.3	180.3	86.7	15.1	Wilmore, unpublished
	male	22.5	179.0	77.3	13.0	(17)
Jockeys	male	30.9	158.2	50.3	14.1	Wilmore, unpublished
Orienteering	male	31.2	—	72.2	16.3	(23)
	female	29.0	—	58.1	18.7	(23)
Pentathlon	female	21.5	175.4	65.4	11.0	(24)
Racketeball	male	25.0	181.7	80.3	8.1	(25)
Rowing						
Heavyweight	male	23.0	192.0	88.0	11.0	(26)
Lightweight	male	21.0	186.0	71.0	8.5	(26)
	female	23.0	173.0	68.0	14.0	(26)
Skiing	male†	25.9	176.6	74.8	7.4	(27)
Alpine	male	21.2	176.0	70.1	14.1	(17)
	male	21.8	177.8	75.5	10.2	(28)
	female	19.5	165.1	58.8	20.6	(28)

Table 5-1. *(Continued)*

Athletic Group or Sport	Sex	Age (yr)	Height (cm)	Weight (kg)	Relative (Fat (%)	Reference
Cross-country	male	21.2	176.0	66.6	12.5	(29)
	male	25.6	174.0	69.3	10.2	(17)
	male	22.7	176.2	73.2	7.9	(28)
	female	24.3	163.0	59.1	21.8	(17)
	female	20.2	163.4	55.9	15.7	(28)
Nordic combination	male	22.9	176.0	70.4	11.2	(17)
	male	21.7	181.7	70.4	8.9	(28)
Skijumping	male	22.2	174.0	69.9	14.3	(17)
Soccer	male	26.0	176.0	75.5	9.6	(30)
Speed skating	male	21.0	181.0	76.5	11.4	(17)
Swimming	male[b]	21.8	182.3	79.1	8.5	(27)
	male[b]	20.6	182.9	78.9	5.0	(12)
	female[b]	19.4	168.0	63.8	26.3	(15)
Sprint	female	—	165.1	57.1	14.6	(31)
Middle distance	female	—	166.6	66.8	24.1	(31)
Distance	female	—	166.3	60.9	17.1	(31)
Tennis	male	—	—	—	15.2	(13)
	male	42.0	179.6	77.1	16.3	(32)
	female	39.0	163.3	55.7	20.3	(32)
Track and field	male[b]	21.3	180.6	71.6	3.7	(12)
	male[b]	—	—	—	8.8	(13)

Runners	male	22.5	177.4	64.5	6.3	(27)
Distance	male	26.1	175.7	64.2	7.5	(33)
	male	26.2	177.0	66.2	8.4	(17)
	male	40-49	180.7	71.6	11.2	(34)
	male	55.3	174.5	63.4	18.0	(35)
	male	50-59	174.7	67.2	10.9	(34)
	male	60-69	175.7	67.1	11.3	(34)
	male	70-75	175.6	66.8	13.6	(34)
	male	47.2	176.5	70.7	13.2	(36)
	female	19.9	161.3	52.9	19.2	(37)
	female	32.4	169.4	57.2	15.2	(38)
Middle distance	male	24.6	179.0	72.3	12.4	(17)
Sprint	female	20.1	164.9	56.7	19.3	(37)
	male	46.5	177.0	74.1	16.5	(35)
Discus	male	28.3	186.1	104.7	16.4	(39)
	male	26.4	190.8	110.5	16.3	Wilmore, unpublished
	female	21.1	168.1	71.0	25.0	(37)
Jumpers and hurdlers	female	20.3	165.9	59.0	20.7	(37)
Shot put	male	27.0	188.2	112.5	16.5	(39)
	male	22.0	191.6	126.2	19.6	(40)
	female	21.5	167.6	78.1	28.0	(37)
Volleyball	female	19.4	166.0	59.8	25.3	(15)
	female	19.9	172.2	64.1	21.3	(41)

Table 5-1. ***(Continued)***

Athletic Group or Sport	Sex	Age (yr)	Height (cm)	Weight (kg)	Relative (Fat (%)	Reference
Weight lifting	male	24.9	166.4	77.2	9.8	(27)
Power	male	26.3	176.1	92.0	15.6	(39)
Olympic	male	25.3	177.1	88.2	12.2	(39)
Body builders	male	29.0	172.4	83.1	8.4	(39)
	male	27.6	178.8	88.1	8.3	(42)
Wrestling	male	26.0	177.8	81.8	9.8	(39)
	male	27.0	176.0	75.7	10.7	(43)
	male	22.0	—	—	5.0	(21)
	male	23.0	—	79.3	14.3	(44)
	male	19.6	174.6	74.8	8.8	(45)
	male	15-18	172.3	66.3	6.9	(46)
	male	20.6	174.8	67.3	4.0	(47)

[a]Reproduced with permission, J. H. Wilmore (11).
[b]Specific events were not specified.

the protein needs of those athletes involved in sports which require training to increase either strength or muscle mass, or both, where actual increases in the contractile proteins are known to occur (48,49).

There are two possible pathways by which increased protein intake could influence performance: more efficient use of protein as a major substrate for muscle contraction, and enhanced synthesis of protein in response to strength-type exercise training. Each of these will be discussed briefly, followed by a brief review of those studies in which protein supplementation has been experimentally evaluated.

Approximately 15–20% of the body's potential energy is found in protein, with skeletal muscle providing a major reserve (50). In 1842, von Liebig stated that the primary fuel for muscular contraction was derived from muscle protein, and he suggested that large quantities of meat should be eaten to replenish the supply (51). In the late 1800s, however, it was generally concluded that the body's protein reserve was not the energy source, and that carbohydrates were the only fuel source for working muscle (52,53). Subsequently, it was discovered that exercising muscles can use plasma glucose, muscle glycogen, plasma free fatty acids, and plasma and muscle triglycerides as energy sources (53). Recently, it has been found that with dynamic exercise of an acute nature, there is a reduction in the rate of muscle protein synthesis, while muscle proteolysis may be increased (53). Further, research indicates that amino acids may account for between 5 and 15% of the oxidative metabolism of the working muscle (53). This contribution will vary, depending on the type of exercise, its duration and intensity, the stage of exercise, and the individual's previous diet (53). Lemon and Nagle (50) have concluded that the branched-chain amino acids (glucose-alanine cycle) are the most important amino acids contributing to exercise energy needs. They further state that, although protein (amino acids) is clearly not as important as either carbohydrates or free fatty acids, under some conditions protein may contribute significantly to the total exercise calories. Thus, protein does appear to be an important energy source during exercise, but there is no evidence at this time that increasing protein intake will enhance metabolic efficiency.

The second pathway by which protein supplementation might increase athletic performance is through its potential enhancement of protein synthesis. Strength-type exercise training is used to increase not only muscle strength, but also muscle mass. For certain types of athletes, increased muscle bulk is considered a desirable outcome of training which could facilitate peak performance, for example, American football and throwing events in track and field. In a recent review article, Booth and coworkers (48) note that during the first 2 hours of exercise, rates of both protein synthesis and protein degradation are decreased in working skeletal muscle. After 4–12 hours of continuous work, protein synthesis and degradation are both increased. This response, however, would appear to be dependent on the type of exercise, as there is a very high degree of specificity of response to different types of exercise (54). Booth and coworkers (48) conclude that a change in muscle protein synthesis is more important than a change in degradation for causing adaptive alterations in the level of protein subsequent to muscular exercise. Further, Goldberg and coworkers (55) have proposed that both an increased rate of synthesis and a decreased rate of degradation are responsible for the increase in muscle mass consequent to strength training. The additional influence of protein supplementation on these adaptive responses of protein synthesis and degradation to exercise training has not been established, although it could conceivably enhance protein synthesis (49).

Does protein supplementation enhance athletic or work performance? Horstman (56) has concluded that the average diet in the Western culture provides adequately for the protein needs of the athlete. Even with heavy physical training or work, where energy expenditure may exceed 20.9 MJ (5000 kcal), the diet consumed should provide adequate total protein if the proportion of protein in the total energy consumed is maintained. Although this would appear to be theoretically sound, studies are equivocal relative to the protein intake levels of athletes. Several of these studies will be reviewed. The reader is referred to a recent paper by Haymes (49) for a more comprehensive review of this area of protein supplementation and athletic performance.

The early studies found little or no difference in performance between diets low, normal, and high in protein. Darling and coworkers (57) studied the effects of a low protein diet (53 g/day) on endurance performance, compared with diets containing normal (95–113 g/day and high (151–292 g/day) levels of protein. No differences between diets were found for endurance, serum protein, erythrocyte count, or hemoglobin content. Pitts and coworkers (58) reported no reduction in endurance following a diet low in protein compared to diets of normal and high protein content.

Rasch and Pierson (59) investigated the effects of a 25 g protein supplement on increases in strength and muscle hypertrophy following 6 weeks of strength training. Strength was significantly increased in both the protein supplement and placebo groups, but there were no changes in arm girth or volume in either group. Rasch and coworkers (60) studied the influence of protein supplementation on physical performance in two groups of marines who were undergoing a 4 week physical training program, consisting primarily of weight training, calisthenics, field maneuvers, sports, and running for about 4 hours per day. One group was given 0.69 g of protein/kg of body weight per day whereas the other group received a placebo. No significant differences were noted between the groups for any of the performance variables, which were basically strength and muscular endurance items, or for serum total protein, blood urea nitrogen, or albumin.

Several studies have reported an increased protein requirement with exercise training. Yoshimura and coworkers (61), in a summary of their previous work, demonstrate a very close association between the anemia identified during hard physical training, which they have referred to as sports anemia, and protein intake levels. They reported a decrease in hemoglobin and plasma protein over the course of strenuous training while consuming a diet containing 1.3 g of protein/kg/day. They found that by taking more than 2.0 g protein/kg/day they could prevent this sports anemia. It could also be prevented by changing the protein source from approximately 30% fish protein and 70% vegetable protein, to 57% animal protein, maintaining the protein intake at 1.2–1.3 g/kg/day. They concluded that sports anemia is the result of an osmotic fragility caused by chemical hemolysis.

Studies examining nitrogen balance in exercising subjects have also found evidence that a protein intake of 1.0 g/kg/day may not be adequate. Gontzea and coworkers (62,63) have found negative nitrogen balances in subjects during exercise training with a protein intake of 1.0 g/kg/day, with the major increase in nitrogen excretion occurring through the sweat. Celejowa and Homa (64) reported five of ten weight lifters in negative nitrogen balance with a protein intake of 2 g/kg/day. Laritcheva and coworkers (65) also found that protein intakes of 2 g/kg/day were inadequate to maintain protein balance, when weight lifters were preparing intensely for an important competition.

Marable and coworkers (66) investigated four groups of college men who consumed two levels of protein (0.8 or 2.4 g/kg/day) for 28 days while serving either as controls or as subjects in a weight training program. Urinary nitrogen expressed relative to protein intake decreased significantly in the exercising subjects, and was more pronounced in the group taking 0.8 g/kg/day. They concluded that the decreases in urinary nitrogen for the exercising subjects at both protein levels could account for sufficient extra nitrogen retention to allow for synthesis of approximately 2 kg of lean weight in 28 days. However, the magnitude of decrease required for the low protein intake group suggested that the protein intake of this group was marginal during muscle building exercise. Consolazio and coworkers (67) studied two groups of men consuming two levels of protein (1.4 and 2.8 g/kg/day) during a 40 day experimental period of intense physical training. Although urinary nitrogens were fairly constant across the two groups, and both groups remained in nitrogen balance, only the group on the high protein diet increased lean body mass significantly, that is, 3.3 kg. Although not reported directly in this study, the authors concluded that the additional body protein did not enhance work performance.

Haymes (49), in her comprehensive review of protein and athletic performance, concludes that a protein intake of 1.0 g/kg/day may be inadequate for the diets of athletes in training. Increased protein intake may be important during the early stages of training to support increases in muscle mass, myoglobin, enzyme content, and erythrocyte formation, and the optimal intake during this period may be as low as 1.2 g/kg/day. For weight lifters, or athletes undergoing intense strength training, optimal intake may be as high as 2.0 g/kg/day.

FAT AND CARBOHYDRATE NEEDS

As was mentioned in the previous section, carbohydrates were at one time considered to be the only fuel source for working muscles. Since that time, fat and protein have been identified as major sources of energy, with fat serving as a primary energy source during exercise, providing 25–90% of the total exercise metabolism (68,69). Does fat have special ergogenic properties, and if it does, should fat be supplemented in the diet? First, the body has an ample amount of fat in storage as adipose tissue. A very lean male distance runner who is 5% body fat at 60 kg, will have 3 kg of fat, or the energy equivalent of over 96.4 MJ (23,000 kcal). This would be sufficient fuel to run over eight marathons (26.2 miles or 42 km per marathon). Most athletes have relative body fats considerably above 5% of their total weight (see Table 5-1). Fat is important as an energy source because it represents a considerable reservoir of stored energy and it is relatively easily mobilized. Conversely, carbohydrates have a finite storage capacity as is illustrated in Table 5-2 for the example of a normal 70 kg man in the postabsorptive state (53).

The importance of fat as a substrate is recognized primarily through its role in sparing the use of carbohydrates, which have a finite and a relatively small energy reserve. The more the body can use fat as the primary substrate the more it can protect its limited carbohydrate supply (70).

How can the athlete adapt to rely more on the use of free fatty acids? First, the rate of glycogen use is directly related to the

Table 5-2.

Body Fuels	kg	kcal
Fat from adipose triglyceride	12	110,000
Muscle protein	6	24,000
Glycogen from liver	0.07	280
Glycogen from muscle	0.40	1600
Glucose from body fluids	0.02	80
Free fatty acids from body fluids	0.004	4
	Total	135,964

intensity of exercise (71–73); the greater the intensity, the greater the rate of use. In addition, the greater the intensity of exercise, the greater the proportional contribution of carbohydrates to the total energy demands (5,6). At low levels of exercise such as walking, that is, at 20–30% of the individual's maximal oxygen uptake or aerobic capacity, muscle glycogen use is very low, and free fatty acids are the primary substrate (74). Havel and coworkers (68) reported that approximately 50% of the total energy expenditure is derived from free fatty acid metabolism when subjects are working at 50% of their aerobic capacity.

Second, as the athlete becomes better conditioned aerobically, through cardiorespiratory endurance training, he or she has an increased capacity to oxidize fatty acids, which results in a greater reliance on fat oxidation for energy during work of the same absolute intensity in the trained state (74, 75). This is the result of an enhanced activity of the enzymes for fat degradation (76,77). Saltin (71) exercised five subjects at the same absolute work load before and after a period of physical training, and found a lower respiratory exchange ratio following training, indicating a greater reliance on fat and a sparing of glycogen. Costill and Miller (5) reported that highly trained marathon runners running at 70% of their aerobic capacity for 60 minutes derived over 75% of their energy from fat metabolism.

Third, it has been demonstrated that free fatty acid use is a direct function of plasma free fatty acid concentrations; that is, the higher the plasma levels the greater the use (78). Rennie and

Holloszy (79) have shown that the availability of free fatty acids has a direct inhibitory effect on glucose uptake and glycogen use in well-oxygenated perfused skeletal muscle. Thus, factors that enhance free fatty acid mobilization and oxidation will result in the sparing of glycogen and generally improve endurance performance. Two factors that have been investigated experimentally are heparin and caffeine.

Three studies were published in 1977 reporting elevations in free fatty acids at rest and during exercise with the administration of heparin. Hickson and coworkers (80) gave rats maize oil by stomach tube, and 3 hours later injected heparin to increase plasma free fatty acid levels. The rats with raised free fatty acids were able to exercise approximately 1 hour longer than control animals before reaching exhaustion (181 versus 118 min). Glycogen concentrations in liver and skeletal muscle, and blood glucose levels, decreased at a significantly slower rate in those animals exercising with increased free fatty acid levels. Costill and coworkers (81) had seven men run for 30 minutes on the treadmill at 70% of their aerobic capacity following one of three conditions: 45 minutes after ingesting 75 g of glucose in 300 ml of water; 4.5–5 hours after eating a high fat meal, with 2000 unit heparin injection 30 minutes prior to exercise; and after a 5–6 hour fast, with the subjects acting as their own controls. The elevation of plasma free fatty acids with the high fat diet and heparin injection decreased the rate of muscle glycogen depletion by 40% as compared to the fasting control. Finally, Ahlborg and Hagenfeldt (82) observed leg and splanchnic exchange of free fatty acids and glucose during 90 minutes of cycling following either normal conditions or the administration of heparin. Heparin elicited a marked increase in plasma free fatty acids at rest. During exercise, plasma values were not different between the two conditions; however, free fatty acid uptake in the exercising legs was augmented after heparin administration as a result of an increase in the fractional leg uptake.

With respect to the influence of caffeine on plasma free fatty acid levels, the early work of Bellet and his associates demonstrated that free fatty acid levels were increased by approximately 50% with either coffee or caffeine sodium benzoate (83). In a later study, Bellet and coworkers (84) observed the effect of coffee, decaffeinated coffee, and a control beverage on plasma free fatty acid levels in a group of normal human subjects, compared to the effect of caffeine sodium benzoate. Significant elevations in free fatty acids were observed after the ingestion of both coffee and caffeine sodium benzoate, reaching peak values in 3 or 4 hours.

Although a number of studies have concentrated on the direct effects of caffeine on various aspects of physical performance (85,86) this review will be limited to those that have used caffeine to stimulate free fatty acid mobilization. Costill and coworkers (87) studied the effects of caffeine ingestion on metabolism and performance during prolonged exercise in nine competitive cyclists. The subjects exercised to exhaustion on a cycle ergometer at 80% of their aerobic capacity, after ingesting either decaffeinated coffee or regular coffee (330 mg of caffeine). The subjects were able to work approximately 20% longer following the ingestion of caffeine (90.2 versus 75.5 minutes) owing to a greater rate of lipid metabolism during the caffeine trial. Ivy and coworkers (88) investigated the effects of caffeine and glucose polymer on work production during 2 hours of isokinetic cycling exercise. Caffeine significantly increased work production by 7.4% compared to control conditions and, during the last 70 minutes of the caffeine trial, fat oxidation was elevated 31% and appeared to provide the substrate needed for the increased work production during this period of exercise. Van Handel (86) has recently conducted a comprehensive review of the literature on caffeine as an ergogenic aid and concludes that caffeine administration does enhance endurance performance primarily as a result of alterations in the mobilization and use of carbohydrate and fat. He also suggests that there may be increases in neuronal excitability, possibly reducing the threshold of motor neurons, thereby altering either fiber recruitment patterns or the perception of work, or both.

A major breakthrough in athletic nutrition came in the 1960s when a group of Scandinavian researchers initiated experimental observations of carbohydrate storage and use with prolonged, endurance-type exercise (89). The early studies of Christensen and Hansen (90) had shown that, as the intensity of exercise increased, the relative contribution of carbohydrate as fuel source increased. Following 3 days on a diet low in carbohydrate, exercise time to exhaustion was significantly reduced. Conversely, following 3 days on a diet high in carbohydrate, exercise time to exhaustion was substantially increased (80 min versus 210 min). In the 1960s, the needle biopsy technique was introduced into the field of exercise physiology and athletic nutrition by Bergstrom (91). This allowed investigators to determine actual alterations in muscle glycogen and varying diets, and the influence of differences in muscle glycogen levels on endurance performance.

In what is now considered to be a classic study, Bergstrom and coworkers (92) provided their subjects with three different diets, each for a prescribed period of time. One diet was high in carbohydrates, the second high in fat and protein (low in carbohydrates), and the third was a normal mixed diet; each diet containing the same number of calories. Before starting the diet, the subject depleted his muscle glycogen stores by riding a cycle ergometer to exhaustion at approximately 75% of his maximal aerobic capacity. This was followed by 3 days on the prescribed diet, and then a second ride to exhaustion. Prior to the second ride, a muscle biopsy was obtained to determine glycogen content. The total length of time the subject could ride before reaching exhaustion and the initial glycogen content were as shown in Table 5-3.

These results supported the earlier work of Christensen and Hansen (90) who observed only changes in performance time

Table 5-3.

Diet	Glycogen content (g/100 g wet tissue)	Time to Exhaustion (minutes)
Mixed	1.75	113.6
High fat and protein	0.63	56.9
High carbohydrate	3.31	166.5

with different diets. In addition, the results of Bergstrom and coworkers (92) illustrate the important relationship between muscle glycogen content and endurance capacity. Others have reported similar results, underlining the very important fact that endurance performance is directly related to the muscle glycogen content at the start of the exercise bout (93–97).

Elevated muscle glycogen stores have been associated with improved performance by athletes in several sports (98), for example, distance runners (99), canoeists (98) and cyclists (100). In addition, Jacobs and coworkers (101) have observed muscle glycogen concentrations in top players from an elite soccer team following a regular season match. They found low glycogen levels immediately following the match. Two days after the match the levels were still relatively low, that is, lower than untrained sedentary subjects. Saltin (72) described a study in which a group of soccer players were glycogen depleted before an exhibition match. During the match, film analysis showed that those players who were glycogen depleted covered less ground during the match, and maintained a slower average speed than the control players.

From the above, it is clear that high muscle glycogen levels are important for peak performance of an endurance nature where the athlete is pushed to exhaustion. Maughan and Poole (102) have even demonstrated a substantial improvement in the performance of an anaerobic exercise bout, that is, cycling to exhaustion, at 104% of the subject's aerobic capacity, following a glycogen loading regimen, although it is generally agreed that glycogen loading is of little benefit for endurance events shorter than 60 minutes in length (6). It is, therefore, important to determine the most efficacious manner of elevating muscle glycogen levels, and to identify and then attempt to modify those factors which influence the rate of muscle glycogen use. Addressing the second of these two aspects first, it has been established in the previous discussion that the rate of glycogen use is dependent on the intensity of the exercise (73), the level of physical conditioning (5,72), and the preexercise diet (6,96). In addition, Fink and coworkers (103) have demonstrated a 76% greater muscle glycogen depletion during 75 minutes of exercise in the heat

(41°C, 15% humidity) compared to the same exercise in the cold (9°C, 55% humidity). Sherman (6), through his review of the literature, has demonstrated that glycogen depletion patterns appear to differ with exercise mode, that is, cycle ergometer exercise results in much more substantial muscle glycogen depletion. Costill and coworkers (104) and Gollnick and coworkers (105) have demonstrated that glycogen depletion patterns are specific to the muscle fiber type, with Type I, or slow twitch, muscle fibers demonstrating more complete depletion with endurance exercise. Finally, Costill and Miller (5) discuss the importance of liver as well as muscle glycogen stores relative to exercise performance. Blood-borne glucose serves as a major contributor to the metabolic pool, representing less than 10% of the total muscle oxygen consumption at rest, but increasing to levels approaching 75-90% of the muscle's carbohydrate metabolism during extended periods of endurance exercise. With the liver serving as the major contributor of glucose in the blood, liver glycogen stores become important when considering the total energy pool.

To conclude this section, it is important to discuss how glycogen stores are elevated to provide the optimal levels for peak athletic performance. In one of the earliest studies, Bergstrom and Hultman (106) had their subjects perform one-legged cycling at 75% of their aerobic capacity until the exercising leg was exhausted. This was followed by rest and a 3 day diet high in carbohydrates. Using the muscle biopsy technique, they demonstrated almost total depletion of muscle glycogen in the exercised leg immediately following the work bout. At the end of the 3 day high carbohydrate diet and rest, the exercised leg had more than doubled its muscle glycogen content above its preexhaustive exercise work bout level, whereas the unexercised leg remained unchanged. Thus, glycogen resynthesis was localized to those muscles which had undergone glycogen depletion. Further, resynthesis appeared to result in a substantial overcompensation, that is, much more glycogen was resynthesized than was depleted.

Sherman (6) has described the resynthesis process as biphasic, with a rapid initial response to preexercise levels, and a slower secondary phase to above-normal levels. Piehl (107) has demonstrated that there is a marked storage of glycogen in the muscle during the first 5 hours following a glycogen-depleting exercise bout which is closely related to the carbohydrate intake. However, preexercise values were not reached until 46 hours after the exercise bout. The amount of carbohydrate consumed following the exercise bout is directly related to the subsequent resynthesis; that is, the more carbohydrate consumed, the greater the resulting muscle glycogen level. This has been demonstrated both following cycle ergometer exercise (95,97) and following treadmill exercise (108). There does appear to be an upper limit, however, with carbohydrate intake in excess of 600 g/day resulting in little further increase in muscle glycogen resynthesis (109).

The type of dietary carbohydrate intake following glycogen depletion can also influence the subsequent levels of glycogen resynthesis. Costill and coworkers (109) studied the effect of the type, amount, and the frequency of feeding carbohydrates on muscle glycogen resynthesis following a glycogen depletion run. They found that both complex and simple carbohydrate diets of approximately 3000 kcal resulted in similar muscle glycogen levels 24 hours after exercise. However, 48 hours after exercise the complex carbohydrate diet resulted in significantly higher muscle glycogen levels. Thus, starch-based diets after the initial 24 hour period following exercise should result in relatively larger amounts of muscle glycogen synthesis compared to equivalent glucose-based diets (6).

The pattern of exercise and diet to ensure optimal muscle glycogen loading prior to athletic competition has received considerable attention. Astrand (110) initially proposed the following routine. Approximately 1 week prior to competition the athlete performs an exhaustive training bout in an attempt to deplete the muscle glycogen stores. This is followed by 3 days of light to moderate activity with a diet low in carbohydrate and high in protein and fat. Finally, 3 days prior to competition the athlete is to minimize activity and consume a diet high in carbohydrate. Several variations on this pattern have been shown to be successful in maximally elevating muscle glycogen levels (6). Sherman (6) however, in his critical review of existing dietary/exercise protocols to optimize muscle glycogen storage, concludes that the best method involves a gradual tapering of activity during the 6 days preceding competition, and a diet that is high in carbohydrate (525 g/day) during the final 3 days prior to competition. This eliminates the need for the depletion and the low carbohydrate phases used in previous protocols. He also emphasizes that enhanced muscle glycogen stores will allow an athlete to maintain a high work intensity longer during prolonged aerobic exercise, but will not allow the athlete to work at a faster rate (6).

As a final note, there has been some concern among the medical community regarding the relative safety of high carbohydrate diets used to increase muscle glycogen storage (111). Changes in ST-T wave and chest pain were reported in a 40-year-old male who followed an extreme version of the carbohydrate loading diet (112). Others have demonstrated concern relative to alterations in blood lipid profiles consequent to these high carbohydrate diets (111). Blair and coworkers (111) investigated blood lipid and electrocardiogram responses to carbohydrate loading in 14 men and women runners immediately preceding a marathon race. Ten runners followed the carbohydrate loading diet whereas four consumed their usual diet. The differences between the two groups in electrocardiographic and blood lipid parameters were small and all changes within normal limits. It was concluded that carbohydrate loading had no adverse effects on those variables studied.

VITAMINS AND MINERALS

Historically, massive doses of various vitamins have been taken by certain athletes in hopes of improving their athletic performance (113). Mineral supplementation has occurred to a much lesser extent. The problems and diseases associated with vitamin deficiencies are well documented, but do athletes have vitamin or mineral deficiencies? In the absence of deficiencies, will supplementation of vitamins or minerals above the RDA result in enhanced athletic performance? This section will review the available literature regarding vitamin and mineral supplementation, and their effects on athletic performance.

Vitamins

Of the 13 substances classified as vitamins, only vitamins C, E, and the B-complex vitamins have been extensively investigated relative to their potential for facilitating athletic performance. B-complex vitamins are involved in coenzyme activity with the metabolism of fats and carbohydrates, and in the formation of erythrocytes (49). Although several studies have shown that the supplementation of one, or a combination, of the B-complex vitamins facilitates performance, there is a general consensus that supplementation is of no measurable value relative to the athlete's performance providing there is not a preexisting deficiency (49,113). In studies where the investigators have created a deficiency in one or more of the B-complex vitamins, there is typically a decrement in performance, which is reversed with supplementation of the deficient vitamins (49).

Vitamin C plays an important role in the formation of collagen, a critical protein in connective tissue, and assists in the absorption of iron. It also functions in the metabolic reactions of amino acids, and in the synthesis of catecholamines and the anti-inflammatory corticoids of the adrenal gland (112). Supplementation of vitamin C has produced equivocal findings in those research studies conducted to date. Several studies have reported increased mechanical efficiency on the cycle ergometer (114,115), increased physical working capacity (116), a reduced exercise and recovery heart rate for the same rate of work (115–117), and a reduced oxygen consumption, pulmonary ventilation, and oxygen debt during or following submaximal exercise (115), following supplementation of vitamin C. Conversely, studies have shown no improvement in aerobic capacity, recovery heart rates, submaximal oxygen uptake, and pulmonary ventilation, 50 km ski race performance, cross-country race performance, treadmill run time to exhaustion, and selected performance variables such as shotput, 100 yd dash, and 1 mile run time (49,111) following supplementation. Burry (118) has stated that it is clearly established that with protein and vitamin C deficiency wound healing is slow and inadequate, but that there is no evidence that vitamin C supplementation in the presence of an adequate dietary intake will prevent injury.

Vitamin E has received a great deal of attention over the years, being the focus of numerous newspaper and magazine articles which have suggested a number of medical conditions that may be alleviated by this miracle vitamin (119). Further, there is good reason to believe that a large segment of the population is consuming large, supplementary doses of vitamin E (119). Vitamin E is a fat soluble vitamin that derives most of its activity from alpha-tocopherol. It is postulated to have an important ergogenic effect through its relationship with oxygen use and energy supply. Although several studies have demonstrated that vitamin E supplementation improves treadmill running time to exhaustion (120), aerobic capacity (121–123), and decreased submaximal oxygen uptake and oxygen debt (122), other studies have reported no change in swimming performance, aerobic capacity, heart-rate recovery, or performances on a standardized step test, pull-ups, push-ups, sit-ups, and a one mile run (49,113).

During the past decade, athletes throughout the world have started experimenting with a new substance which has been incorrectly identified as a vitamin, that is, pangamic acid, or vitamin B-15, as it is commonly called. Initial studies from Russia suggested that pangamic acid could increase oxygen use by the muscle tissue and increase the intensity of aerobic oxidation. In addition, pangamic acid was shown to slow the ageing process, assist bone healing, normalize blood sugar metabolism, and lower blood lactate levels (124). Although this has not been studied extensively in the United States, two recent studies have shown that pangamic acid does not produce significant changes in short-term maximal treadmill performance (124), or in short-term submaximal cycle ergometer performance (125).

It appears that in the absence of a specific vitamin deficiency, supplementation with vitamins has little or no benefit relative to enhanced athletic performance. However, many of the previous studies have lacked adequate controls, have not had proper experimental designs, and have used questionable performance parameters. More rigorous studies using proper controls and experimental designs, and more relevant criteria of athletic performance, will be necessary before any final conclusions can be drawn regarding vitamin supplementation and athletic performance.

Minerals

Minerals, unlike vitamins, are much less likely to be supplemented by the athletic population. Far less concern has been shown by the athlete for his or her mineral status, possibly because there have been far fewer ergogenic qualities ascribed to specific minerals. Some attention has been focused on the electrolytes, since sweat rates of 2 1/hour or greater are associated with electrolyte losses. A number of commercial beverages have been developed to assist the athlete in replacing those electrolytes lost during exercise. Costill and Miller (5), however, have shown that the electrolyte loss during exercise is actually very small, even with high rates of sweating, and that these small losses are replaced with a normal dietary intake over the subsequent 24 hour period. In fact, Costill (70) has recommended that an ideal fluid replacement solution should contain few, if any, electrolytes, contain less than 2.5 g of glucose per 100 ml of water, have an osmolality of approximately 200 mOsm/1, be ingested at frequent intervals in volumes of 100 to 200 ml, and be cold (4°C).

Of the remaining minerals, iron and calcium have been most frequently investigated. Unfortunately, only a few studies have been conducted on calcium supplementation, but these would suggest supplementation is of no value in the presence of a normal dietary calcium intake. Iron, however, has received a great deal of attention in the research literature. First, it has been estimated that 22% of females in the United States, 17 to 44 years of age, with hemoglobin levels above 10 g/100 ml are iron deficient (126). Further, in a study of male and female middle and long distance runners, Clement and Asmundson (127) reported that 29% of the men and 82% of the women had plasma ferritin concentrations at risk for iron deficiency. Ehn and coworkers (128) in their study of 8 male long distance runners, found normal hemoglobin and serum iron levels, but bone marrow studies showed either an absence, or only traces, of iron, indicating latent iron deficiency. They attributed this deficiency to a low absorption and an increased elimination of iron. Hunding and coworkers (129) identified iron deficiency in 63 of 113 joggers and competitive runners, with 13 of the women and 10 of the men demonstrating latent anemia. Oral iron therapy normalized the hemoglobin concentrations, and led to the establishment of personal records for the competitive runners.

Recent reviews (49,113,130) have reported the incidence of iron deficiency among athletes from various populations. Studies generally suggest that 22–25% of female athletes and 10% of male athletes are iron deficient. When iron supplements are given to those who are iron deficient, performance measures are typically improved, particularly aerobic capacity (49,113,130). However, supplementation of iron in those who are not deficient appears to have no benefit (49,113).

We have attempted to collate the available research on the role of nutrition in optimizing athletic performance. By necessity, discussion has been limited in breadth of topic areas as well as in depth of coverage. The reader is referred to the reviews published over the past ten years, referenced in specific sections of this paper, for a more detailed discussion and list of references. Further, discussion in this area is also limited by the difficulty of designing studies to answer the questions that need to be answered. Athletes are very complex models to study. By their very nature they are unique, not representing the normal population, and they are greatly influenced by psychological as well as physiological factors. Often, denying the athlete a certain food that he or she associates with success, will result in the total failure of that athlete, irrespective of the scientific merits of the food in question. These factors must be considered as the next generation of experiments reach the planning stages. Proper questions must be asked, and the evaluative criteria must be appropriate for those questions. Experimental designs must be improved, assuring adequate controls. Finally, statistical procedures must be carefully selected, for a 1–2% improvement may not reach statistical significance, but it may mean the difference between winning the gold as opposed to the silver medal.

This review has demonstrated that nutrition plays an important part in optimizing athletic performance. In most cases, however, adequate dietary intake of the essential foods, vitamins, and minerals is all that is necessary, without the need for supplementation. Although this statement would seem to stand on its own merit, it is also important to point out that most athletes have little or no idea what it means to eat a good, nutritionally sound, diet. Thus, education and example must be the cornerstone of any effort to improve the athlete's performance potential through sound nutritional practices.

REFERENCES

1. G. E. Butterfield, "Fats, Carbohydrates, and Protein: Why We Need Them, and How They Are Obtained," in W. Haskell, J. Scala, and J. Whittam, Eds., *Nutrition and Athletic Performance,* Bull Publishers, Palo Alto, 1982, pp. 2–15.
2. N. J. Smith, *Food for Sport,* Bull Publishers, Palo Alto, 1976, pp. 1–169.
3. M. H. Williams, *Nutrition for Fitness and Sport,* Wm. C. Brown, Dubuque, Iowa, 1983, pp. 1-296.
4. J. H. Wilmore, Training for Sport and Activity: *The Psysiological Basis of the Conditioning Process,* 2nd ed., Allyn and Bacon, Boston, 1982, pp. 167–184.
5. D. L. Costill and J. M. Miller, *Int. J. Sports Med.,* **1,** 2 (1980).
6. W. M. Sherman, "Carbohydrates, Muscle Glycogen, and Muscle Glycogen Supercompensation," in M. H. Williams, Ed., *Ergogenic Aids in Sport,* Human Kinetics, Champaign, Il., 1983, pp. 3–26.
7. P. O. Astrand, "Nutrition and Physical Performance," in M. Rechcigl, Jr., Ed., *Nutrition and the World Food Problem,* S. Karger, Basel, 1979, pp. 63-84.
8. C. M. Tipton, "Consequences of Rapid Weight Loss," in W. Haskell, J. Scala, and J. Whittam, Eds., *Nutrition and Athletic Performance,* Bull Publishers, Palo Alto, 1982, pp. 176–197.
9. G. R. Leon, *Med. Sci. Sports Exerc.,* **15,** 89 (1983).
10. C. Lentner, Ed., *Geigy Scientific Tables, Volume I. Units of Measurement, Body Fluids, Composition of the Body, Nutrition,* Ciba-Geigy, Switzerland, 1981, pp. 232–234.
11. J. H. Wilmore, *Med. Sci. Sports Exerc.,* **15,** 21 (1983).
12. L. P. Novak, R. E. Hyatt, and J. F. Alexander, *J.A.M.A.,* **205,** 764 (1968).
13. H. L. Forsyth and W. E. Sinning, *Med. Sci. Sports Exerc.,* **5,** 174 (1973).

14. W. E. Sinning, *Res. Quart.*, **44,** 313 (1973).
15. P. R. Conger, and R. B. J. Macnab, *Res. Quart.*, **38,** 184 (1967).
16. R. B. Parr, J. H. Wilmore, R. Hoover, D. Bachman, and R. Kerlan, *Physician Sportsmed.*, **6,** 77 (1978).
17. Rusko, M. Hara, L. *Eur. J. Appl. Physiol.*, 151 (1978).
18. J. D., Wickkiser and J. M. Kelly, *Med. Sci. Sports Exerc.*, **7,** 199 (1975).
19. J. H. Wilmore, R. B. Parr, W. L. Haskell, D. L. Costill, L. J. Milburn, and R. K. Kerlan, *Physician Sportsmed.*, **4,** 45 (1976).
20. W. E. Sinning and G. D. Lindberg, *Res. Quart.*, **43,** 226 (1972).
21. J. Parizkova, "Body Composition and Exercise during Growth and Development," in G. L. Rarick, Ed., *Physical Activity, Human Growth and Development.* Academic, New York, 1973, pp. 97-124.
22. J. Parizkova and O. Poupa, "Some metabolic consequences of adaptation to muscular work," *Bri. J. Nutr.*, **17,** 341 (1963).
23. R. G. Knowlton, K. J. Ackerman, P. I. Fitzgerald, S. W. Wilde, and M. V. Tahamont, *Med. Sci. Sports Exerc.*, **12,** 164 (1980).
24. G. S. Krahenbuhl, C. L. Wells, C. H. Brown, and P. E. Ward, *Med. and Sci. Sports Exerc.*, **11,** 20 (1979).
25. T. V. Pipes, *Physician and Sportsmed.*, **7,** 91 (1979).
26. F. C. Hagerman, G. R. Hagerman, and T. C. Mickelson, *Physician and Sportsmed.*, **7,** 74 (1979).
27. S. Sprynarova and J. Parizkova, *Int. Zeir Angewandte Physiol.*, **29,** 184 (1971).
28. E. M. Haymes, and A. L. Dickinson, *Med. Sci. Sports Exerc.*, **12,** 153 (1980).
29. V. Niinimaa, M. Dyon, and J. F. Alexander, *Med. Sci. Sports Exerc.*, **10,** 91 (1978).
30. P. B. Raven, L. R. Gettman, M. L. Pollock, and K. H. Cooper, *Brit. J. Sports Med.*, **10,** 209 (1976).
31. J. H. Wilmore, C. H. Brown, and J. A. Davis, *Ann. N. Y. Acad. Sci.*, **301,** 764 (1977).
32. P. A. Vodak, W. M. Savin, W. L. Haskell, and P. D. Wood, *Med. Sci. Sports Exerc.*, **12,** 159 (1980).
33. D. L. Costill, R. Bowers, and W. F. Kammer, *Med. Sci. Sports Exerc.*, **2,** 93 (1970).
34. M. L. Pollock, H. S. Miller, and J. Wilmore, *J. Gerontol.*, **29,** 645 (1974).
35. R. J. Barnard, G. K. Grimditch, and J. H. Wilmore, *Med. Sci. Sports Exerc.*, **11,** 167 (1979).
36. S. Lewis, W. L. Haskell, H. Klein, J. Halpern, and P. D. Wood, *J. Appl. Physiol.*, **39,** 221 (1975).
37. R. M. Malina, A. B. Harper, H. H. Avent, and D. E. Campbell, *Med. Sci. Sports Exerc.*, **3,** 32 (1971).
38. J. H. Wilmore and C. H. Brown, *Med. Sci. Sports Exerc.*, **6,** 178 (1974).
39. T. D. Fahey, L. Akka, R. Rolph, *J. Appl. Physiol.*, **39,** 559 (1975).
40. A. R. Behnke, and J. H. Wilmore, *Evaluation and Regulation of Body Build and Composition,* Prentice Hall, Englewood Cliffs, N.J., 1974.

41. J. E. Kovaleski, R. B. Parr, J. E. Hornak, and J. L. Roitman, *Physician and Sportsmed.*, **8**, 112 (1980).
42. T. V. Pipes, *Physician and Sportsmed.*, **7**, 116 (1979).
43. J. B. Gale and K. W. Flynn, *Med. Sci. Sports Exerc.*, **6**, 232 (1974).
44. A. W. Taylor, L. Brassard, L. Proten, and D. Robin, *Cana. J. Appl. Sport Sci.*, **4**, 131 (1979).
45. W. E. Sinning, *Med. Sci. Sports Exerc.*, **6**, 139 (1974).
46. F. I. Katch, E. D. Michael, and E. M. Jones, *Med. Sci. Sports Exerc.*, **3**, 190 (1971).
47. G. Stine, R. Ratliff, G. Shierman, W. A. Grara, *Physician and Sportsmed.*, **7**, 98 (1979).
48. F. W. Booth, W. F. Nicholson, and P. A. Watson, "Influence of Muscle Use on Protein Synthesis and Degradation," in R. L. Terjung, Ed., *Exercise and Sport Sciences Reveiws, Vol. 10,* Franklin Institute, Philadelphia, 1982, pp. 27-48.
49. E. M. Haymes, "Proteins, Vitamins, and Iron," in M. H. Williams, Ed., *Ergogenic Aids in Sport,* Human Kinetics, Champaign, Il, 1983, pp. 27–55.
50. P. W. R. Lemon and F. J. Nagle, *Med. Sci. Sports Exerc.*, **13**, 141 (1981).
51. J. vonLiebig, *Animal Chemistry and Its Application to Physiology and Pathology,* Taylor and Walton, London, 1842.
52. A. Chauveau, *Comptes Rendus (Paris),* **122**, 1163 (1896).
53. M. N. Goodman and N. B. Ruderman, Influence of muscle use on amino acid metabolism, in R. L. Terjung, Ed., *Exercise and Sport Sciences Reviews, Vol. 10,* Franklin Institute, Philadelphia, 1982, pp. 1–26.
54. J. O. Holloszy and F. W. Booth, *Ann. Rev. Physiol.*, **38**, 223 (1976).
55. A. L. Goldberg, J. D. Etlinger, D. F. Goldspink, and C. Jablecki, *Med. Sci. Sports Exerc.*, **7**, 185 (1975).
56. D. H. Horstman, "Nutrition," in W. P. Morgan, Ed., *Ergogenic Aids and Muscular Performance,* Academic, New York, 1972, pp. 343-365.
57. R. C. Darling, R. E. Johnson, G. C. Pitts, F. C. Consolazio, and P. F. Robinson, *J. Nutrition,* **28**, 273 (1944).
58. G. C. Pitts, F. C. Consolazio, and R. E. Johnson, *J. Nutrition,* **27**, 497 (1944).
59. P. J. Rasch and W. R. Pierson, *Am. J. Clin. Nutr.*, **11**, 530 (1962).
60. P. J. Rasch, J. W. Hamby, and H. J. Burns, *Med. Sci. Sports Exerc.*, **1**, 195 (1969).
61. H. Yoshimura, T. Inoue, T. Yamada, and K. Shiraki, *World Rev. Nutr. Dietetics,* **35**, 1 (1980).
62. I. Gontzea, P. Sutzescu, and S. Dumitrache, *Nutr. Rep. Internat.*, **10**, 35 (1974).
63. I. Gontzea, R. Sutzescu, and S. Dumitrache, *Nutr. Repts. Internatl.*, **11**, 231 (1975).
64. I. Celejowa and M. Homa, *Nutr. and Metab.*, **12**, 259 (1970).
65. K. A. Laritcheva, N. I. Yalovaya, V. I. Shubin, and P. V. Smirnov, "Study of Energy Expenditure and Protein Needs of Top Weight Lifters," in J. Parizkova and V. A. Rogozkin, Eds., *Nutrition, Physical Fitness, and Health,* University Park Press, Baltimore, pp. 155–163.

66. N. L. Marable, J. F. Hickson, M. K. Korslund, W. G. Herbert, R. F. Desjardins, and F. W. Thye, *Nutr. Repts Internatl,* **19,** 795 (1979).
67. C. F. Consolazio, H. L. Johnson, R. A. Nelson, J. G. Dramise, and J. H. Skala, *Am. J. Clin. Nutr.,* **28,** 29 (1975).
68. R. J. Havel, A. Naimark, and C. R. Borchgrevin, *J. Clin. Invest.,* **42,** 1054 (1963).
69. L. A. Carlson, L.-G. Eklund, and L. Oro, *J. Lab. Clin. Med.,* **61,** 724 (1963).
70. D. L. Costill, "A Scientific Approach to Distance Running," *Track and Field News,* Los Altos, 1979, pp. 1-128.
71. B. Essen, *Ann. N.Y. Acad. Sci.,* **301,** 30 (1977).
72. B. Saltin, *Med. Sci. Sports Exerc.,* **5,** 137 (1973).
73. B. Saltin and J. Karlsson, *Adv. Exp. Med. Biol.,* **11,** 289 (1971).
74. P. D. Gollnick, *Ann. N.Y. Acad. Sci.,* **301,** 64 (1977).
75. J. O. Holloszy, M. J. Rennie, R. C. Hickson, R. K. Conlee, J. M. Hagberg, *Ann. N.Y. Acad. Sci.,* **301,** 440 (1977).
76. J. O. Holloszy, L. B. Oscal, I. J. Don, and P. A. Mole, *Biochem. Biophys. Res. Comm.,* **40,** 1368 (1970).
77. P. A. Mole and J. O. Holloszy, *Pro. Soc. Exptl. Biol. Med.,* **134,** 789 (1970).
78. R. J. Havel, B. Pernow, and N. L. Jones, *J. Appl. Physiol.,* **23,** 90 (1966).
79. M. J. Rennie and J. O. Holloszy, *Biochem. J.,* **168,** 161 (1977).
80. R. C. Hickson, M. J. Rennie, R. K. Conlee, W. W. Winder, and J. O. Holloszy, *Appl. Physiol.: Resp. Environ. Exercise Physiol.,* **43,** 829 (1977).
81. D. L. Costill, E. Coyle, G. Dalsky, W. Evans, W. Fink, and D. Hoopes, *J. Appl. Physiol.: Resp. Environ. Exercise Physiol.,* **43,** 695 (1977).
82. G. Ahlborg and L. Hagenfeldt, *Scand. J. Clin. Lab. Invest.,* **37,** 619 (1977).
83. S. Bellet, A. Kershbaum, and J. Aspe, *Arch. Int. Med.,* **116,** 750 (1965).
84. S. Bellet, A. Kershbaum, and E. M. Finck, *Metabolism,* **17,** 702 (1968).
85. R. Perkins and M. H. Williams, *Med. Sci. Sports Exerc.,* **7,** 221 (1975).
86. P. Van Handel, "Caffeine," in M. H. Williams, Ed., *Ergogenic Aids in Sport,* Human Kinetics, Champaign, Ill., 1983, pp. 128-163.
87. D. L. Costill, G. P. Dalsky, and W. J. Fink, *Med. Sci. Sports Exerc.,* **10,** 155 (1978).
88. J. L. Ivy, D. L. Costill, W. J. Fink, and R. W. Lower, *Med. Sci. Sports Exerc.,* **11,** 6 (1979).
89. J. Bergstrom and E. Hultman, *J.A.M.A.,* **221,** 999 (1972).
90. E. H. Christensen and O. Hansen, *Scand. Arch. of Physiol.,* **81,** 160 (1939).
91. J. Bergstrom, *Scand. J. Clin. Lab. Invest.,* **14,** Suppl. 68 (1962).
92. J. Bergstrom, L. Hermansen, E. Hultman, B. Saltin, *Acta Physiol. Scand.,* **71,** 140 (1967).
93. J. Bergstrom and E. Hultman, *Scand. J. Clin. Lab. Invest.,* **19,** 218 (1967).
94. L. Hermansen, E. Hultman, and B. Saltin, *Acta Physiol. Scand.,* **71,** 129 (1967).
95. E. Hultman, *Scand. J. Clin. Lab. Invest.,* **19,** Suppl. 94 (1967).
96. B. Martin, S. Robinson, and D. Robertshaw, *Am. J. Clin. Nutr.,* **31,** 62 (1978).

97. B. Saltin and L. Hermansen, "Glycogen Stores and Prolonged Severe Exercise," in G. Blix, Ed., *Nutrition and Physical Activity.* Almqvist & Wiksells, Uppsala, Sweden, 1967, pp. 32-46.
98. J. V. G. A. Durnin, *Int. J. Sports Med.,* **3,** 52 (1982).
99. J. Karlsson and B. Saltin, *J. Appl. Physiol.,* **31,** 203 (1971).
100. J. D. Brooke, G. J. Davies, and L. F. Green, *J. Sports Med. and Physical Fitness,* **15,** 257 (1975).
101. I. Jacobs, N. Westlin, J. Karlsson, M. Rasmusson, and B. Houghton, *J. Appl. Physiol. Occupational Physiol.,* **48,** 297 (1982).
102. R. J. Maughan and D. C. Poole, *Eur. J. of Appl. Physiol. and Occupational Physiol.,* **46,** 211 (1981).
103. W. J. Fink, D. L. Costill, and P. J. Van Handel, *Eur. J. Appl. Physiol. and Occupational Physiol.,* **34,** 183 (1975).
104. D. L. Costill, P. D. Gollnick, E. D. Jansson, B. Saltin, and E. M. Stein, *Acta Physiol. Scand.,* **89,** 374 (1973).
105. P. D. Gollnick, K. Piehl, C. W. Saubert, IV, R. B. Armstrong, and B. Saltin, *J. Appl. Physiol.,* **33,** 421 (1972).
106. J. Bergstrom and E. Hultman, *Nature,* **210,** 309 (1967).
107. K. Piehl, *Acta Physiol. Scand.,* **90,** 297 (1974).
108. D. L. Costill, P. Blom, and L. Hermansen, *Med. Sci. Sports Exerc.,* **13,** 90 (abstract) (1981).
109. D. L. Costill, W. M. Sherman, W. J. Fink, C. Maresh, M. Witten, and J. M. Miller, *Am. J. Clin. Nutr.,* **34,** 1831 (1981).
110. P.-O. Astrand, *Fed. Proceed.,* **26,** 1772 (1967).
111. S. Blair, R. Sargent, D. Davidson, and R. Krejci, *Physician Sportsmed.,* **8,** 68 (1980).
112. G. Mirkin, *J.A.M.A.,* **223,** 1511 (1973).
113. M. H. Williams, (1982). "Vitamin, Iron and Calcium Supplementation: Effect on Human Physical Performance," in W. Haskell, J. Scala, and J. Whittam, Eds., *Nutrition and Athletic Performance,* Bull Publishing, Palo Alto, 1982, pp. 106-153.
114. A. Hoogerwerf and A. W. J. H. Hoitink, *Int. Zeir Angewandte Physiol.,* **20,** 164 (1963).
115. F. Spioch, R. Kobza, and B. Mazur, *Acta Physiol. Polonica,* **17,** 251 (1966).
116. H. Howald and B. Segesser, *Ann. N. Y. Acad. Sci.,* **258,** 458 (1975).
117. W. Van Huss, *Nutrition Today,* **1,** 20 (1966).
118. H. C. Burry, "Soft Tissue Injury in Sport," in J. H. Wilmore and J. F. Keogh, *Exercise and Sport Sciences Reviews, Vol. 3, Academic, New York, 1975, pp. 275-301.*
119. P. M. Farrell and J. G. Bieri, *Am. J. Clin. Nutr.,* **28,** 1381 (1975).
120. T. Cureton, *Scholastic Coach,* **24,** 36 (1955).
121. D. Clausen, "The Combined Effect of Aerobic Exercise and Vitamin E upon Cardiorespiratory Endurance and Measured Blood Variables." *Unpublished masters thesis.* University of Wyoming, 1971.
122. Y. Kobayashi, "Effect of Vitamin E on Aerobic Work Performance in Man

during Acute Exposure to Hypoxic Hypoxia." *Unpublished doctoral dissertation,* University of New Mexico, 1974.

123. T. Nagawa, *Asian Med. J.*, **11**, 619-633 (1968).
124. M. E. Gray and L. W. Titlow, *Med. Sci. Sports Exerc.*, **14**, 424 (1982).
125. R. N. Girandola, R. A. Wiswell, and R. Bulbulian, *Biochem. Med.*, **24**, 218 (1980).
126. Ten States Nutrition Survey (1972), *Ten States Nutrition Survey 1968-1970: IV Biochemical,* Department of Health, Education and Welfare Pubs. No. (HMS) 72-8132.
127. D. B. Clement and R. C. Asmundson, *Physician and Sportsmed.*, **10**, 37 (1982).
128. L. Ehn, B. Carlmark, and S. Hoglund, *Med. Sci. Sports Exerc.*, **12**, 61 (1980).
129. A. Hunding, R. Jordal, and P.-E. Paulev, *Acta Med. Scand.*, **209**, 315 (1981).
130. R. R. Pate, *Physician Sportsmed.*, **11**, 115 (1983).

6

Special Concerns for Exercise in Women

MONA M. SHANGOLD, M.D.

Georgetown University School of Medicine, Washington, D.C.

Exercise is more important for women than for men and becomes increasingly important for women as they get older. Women are more susceptible than men to both osteoporosis and obesity, the latter of which is associated with increased risks of heart disease, diabetes mellitus, and certain cancers. Regular exercise can prevent both osteoporosis and obesity and their complications.

It is more difficult to acquire the regular habit in later years if a sedentary lifestyle had been followed previously. It is much easier to attain and maintain the practice of regular exercise throughout life if the habits were acquired in youth.

YOUNG GIRLS

Girls who exercise strenuously prior to puberty are more likely to experience menarche at a later age than their sedentary peers (1,2). However, this menarcheal delay is associated with no medical problems, despite possible psychological hazards.

It remains unclear whether exercise delays menarche by promoting thinness or menarcheal delay contributes to athletic success and perseverance by promoting tallness and thinness. Probably both factors are contributory.

Any girl who reaches the age of fourteen without experiencing any secondary sexual development should be examined by a physician, who will determine whether further evaluation is indicated. Any girl who has not begun to menstruate by the age of sixteen should be examined by a gynecologist, who will determine whether further evaluation and treatment are indicated. The exercise is desirable and should be continued during evaluation and treatment.

MENSTRUAL IRREGULARITY AND AMENORRHEA

Menstrual irregularity and amenorrhea are more prevalent among athletes (20%) than among the general population (5%) (3). The many factors which change during the course of a regular training program make it difficult to pinpoint causality. Most women lose weight and fat when they begin to exercise regularly, particularly when they engage in aerobic exercise. Weight loss alone can lead to amenorrhea (4), even in the absence of exercise. Thinness, too, is associated with amenorrhea, even in the absence of exercise (3). Physical stress can contribute to the problem, and emotional stress, which is more difficult to quantify, may also play a role. Amenorrheic runners tend to associate more stress with their running than do regularly menstruating runners (5).

Any insult to the reproductive system of a woman leads to an orderly sequence of dysfunction, and the same pattern is seen in athletes who develop menstrual dysfunction: short luteal phase (the portion of the cycle following ovulation), euestrogenic anovulation (lack of ovulation in women producing normal amounts of estrogen), and hypoestrogenic amenorrhea (absence of menstruation in women producing inadequate amounts of estrogen).

The first abnormality a woman usually develops when she begins to exercise heavily is shortening of the luteal phase, accompanied by less progesterone production in that portion of the cycle (6). This may lead to infertility and requires treatment only when it does so.

The next abnormality a woman usually develops with increasing exercise is one in which ovulation does not occur, but she continues to produce adequate amounts of estrogen. Such a woman does not make progesterone. Since estrogen stimulates the inner lining of the uterus to grow, and since progesterone protects it from overgrowth, the lack of progesterone increases the risks of such women for developing uterine cancer and breast cancer (7).

The next abnormality, which is the most serious one, is one in which the woman makes inadequate amounts of both estrogen and progesterone. This increases her risks of developing both osteoporosis and vaginal dryness (8).

Any women with these menstrual problems should be thoroughly evaluated in the same manner effected for nonathletes with these problems. Blood concentrations of the following hormones should be measured and should be further investigated if abnormal: prolactin, thyroxine, T_3 resin uptake, thyrotropin, follicle stimulating hormone, and luteinizing hormone. It can be determined whether a woman is producing estrogen or not by testing her with a progesterone challenge. Any woman whose uterus has been stimulated by estrogen will have withdrawal bleeding following administration of progesterone; lack of withdrawal bleeding following progesterone administration indicates lack of estrogen stimulation of the uterus.

Women who are deficient in the hormone progesterone should be treated with monthly progesterone, to protect their uteri and breasts. Women who are deficient in both estrogen and progesterone should be treated with both of these hormones, in order to protect their bones.

PREGNANCY

Pregnant women who are accustomed to regular aerobic exercise can continue such exercise as long as their pregnancies are normal and without complications. Aerobic exercises should not be initiated during pregnancy by women who have not practiced them consistently before.

Pregnant women should avoid hyperthermia, which may result during exercise, since hyperthermia in early pregnancy is associated with an increased risk of birth defects and in later pregnancy is associated with an increased risk of premature labor.

Weight lifting and calisthenics are fine exercises for pregnant women, even if they have not practiced them before.

CONTRACEPTION

More runners use the diaphragm for contraception than any other method (3). However, the choice of an athlete's contraceptive method should rarely be affected by the fact that she exercises.

OLDER WOMEN

Because of the increased risks of osteoporosis, obesity, heart disease, diabetes, and depression among older women, exercise is even more important for older women than for younger women. The most effective way for a woman to preserve bone density is by consuming adequate dietary calcium, engaging in regular exercise (particularly weight-bearing exercises), and by maintaining a normal estrogen level. Older women should discuss estrogen replacement therapy with their gynecologists.

REFERENCES

1. R. M. Malina, *Med. Sci. Sports,* **5,** 11 (1973).
2. M. Warren, *J. Clin. Endocrinol. Metab.,* **51,** 1150 (1980).
3. M. M. Shangold and H. S. Levine, *Am. J. Obstet. Gynecol.,* **143,** 862 (1982).
4. A. C. Wentz, *Obstet. Gynecol.,* **56,** 482 (1980).

5. B. Schwartz, D. C. Cumming, E. Riordan, S. S. C. Yen, and R. W. Rebar, *Am. J. Obstet. Gynecol.*, **141,** 662 (1981).
6. M. Shangold, R. Freeman, B. Thysen, and M. Gatz, *Fertil. Steril.*, **31,** 130 (1979).
7. C. B. Coulam, J. F. Annegers, and J. S. Kranz, *Obstet. Gynecol.*, **61,** 403 (1983).
8. S. Meema and H. E. Meema, *Isr. J. Med. Sci.*, **12,** 601 (1976).

7

Special Considerations of Exercise in Children and Adolescents

ODED BAR-OR, M.D.

McMaster University, Hamilton, Ontario, Canada

Most knowledge of the physiologic responses of humans to exercise is based on research with young adults, notably college students or soldiers. Far less information is based on research done with children and adolescents. Interest in pediatric exercise physiology has increased in the last 10 to 15 years, along with the growing participation of children and adolescents in elite sports. Concurrently, there has been an increasing awareness among health professionals of the clinical relevance of exercise to pediatric diagnosis and management.

Some principles of study design, exercise testing, or exercise prescription are valid for any age group. Others must take into account the body size, body proportions, stage of maturation, and mental age of the population in question. This chapter highlights such special considerations, in the study of children's response to exercise and in the clinical implications of exertion for pediatric populations.

The following is not a comprehensive review of pediatric exercise physiology but rather an overview of arbitrarily selected topics, which reflect my special interests. More systematic information on the response of children to exercise can be found in proceedings of symposia of the International Group of Pediatric Work Physiology (1–8), monographs (9–11), recently edited volumes (12–14), and an edited report (15).

METHODOLOGY OF EXERCISE TESTING

Both technical and ethical issues must be considered in the selection and execution of exercise tests of children.

Technical Considerations

The Ergometer. When maximal aerobic power is sought, treadmill running or walking will yield higher maximal oxygen uptake than cycling. While this is true for any age group, it is especially so in young children, probably because of the relatively small mass of their thigh muscles. Children as young as 4 years of age can master the walking or running technique on the treadmill. When using a cycle ergometer, attention must be paid to the small size of the child. Few children under 8 years can use an adult-size ergometer. As pediatric ergometers are seldom produced (one successful attempt has been made by Monark, Sweden), one may have to resort to adaptation of adult-size ergometers.

In addition to lowering the seat one must shorten the pedal crank. A crank length of 9 cm (compared with 17.5 cm in ergometers for adults) has been found in our laboratory to suit most 4 to 5 year old children. Klimt and Voigt (16) found that, for 6 year old children, pedaling a 13 cm crank is metabolically more economical than using a 10 or 18 cm crank. Other modifications include lengthening of the handlebar and allowing the seat to move forwards or backwards. Modifications along the same line must be made in arm ergometers.

Other Apparatus. When expired gas is collected, the dead space of the system must be kept small. Special attention must be given to the mouthpiece and the three-way valve, the combined dead space of which should not exceed 50 ml (9). An adult-size mouthpiece is often uncomfortably large for children. One solution is to cut the edges of the mouth portion.

Some ingenuity is needed in the construction of a metronome for children. While some can follow the common pendulum metronome, others may need such feedback as moving lights (available in the Swiss-made Fleisch-Metabo ergometer) or computer-based animation. Further research and development are needed in this area.

Protocols. In general, exercise testing protocols can be similar in children and adults. One consideration is the total duration of the aerobic power test: because of their short attention span, children should be given tests that do not last more than 8–10 minutes. This duration can be achieved in a progressively increasing protocol by a careful selection of the initial load.

To study physiologic function during submaximal exercise one must know when a steady state has been reached. Some (17), but not all (Cooper, personal communication), studies suggest that children reach a steady state faster than adults. Skinner and coworkers (18) have shown that for 6 to 15 year old girls and boys, 2 minute stages in a progressive-continuous protocol yields the same submaximal and maximal results as 3 minute or 4 minute stages. Anaerobic power can be reliably assessed using the 30 second Wingate test (19). For a review of exercise protocols for children see Bar-Or (11).

Fitness Indices. When analyzing age-related differences in exercise performance, one must be cautious in selecting fitness indices. The use of submaximal heart rate for assessment of maximal aerobic power (whether for prediction of maximal oxygen uptake or as W_{170}) should be limited to population studies and not used to analyze individual changes. This is because of the low correlation between data obtained from submaximal heart rate and those derived from direct determination of maximal O_2 uptake (20,21). The rationale for using W_{170} to compare aerobic fitness across ages is questionable because any given submaximal heart rate in children denotes a lower physiologic strain than it does in adolescents or adults (22,23). If one *must* resort to submaximal protocols, due attention must be given to habituating the subjects.

Furthermore, in using submaximal heart rate as a criterion of aerobic fitness one assumes a certain maximal heart rate. Whereas maximal heart rate of most healthy children ranges between 195 and 205 beat/minute, it may be well below age-appropriate levels in such diseases as anorexia nervosa (24), congenital complete heart block (25), other congenital heart diseases (26,27), or diseases with muscle wasting (28). A child with congenital complete heart block, for example, will have low ventricular rate at rest and at any exercise level (25,29,30). This may lead to a marked overestimation of his maximal aerobic power, whereas in reality this child cannot sufficiently raise his cardiac output during exercise, and his maximal aerobic power is subnormal.

Field tests for determination of maximal aerobic power have their own pitfalls. Such tests as the 12 or 8 minute run/walk assume that the individual performs at his best. This requires pacing and motivation. While children can become motivated to perform an "all-out" task it is hard for them to find the optimal pace unless they have gained some experience in competitive running. Such field tests will particularly underestimate performance of the inexperienced unfit child.

Habituation. To many children, the first encounter with an exercise laboratory may be an emotion-laden experience. This may affect their performance, as well as some of their physiologic responses (31). Heart rate, for example, may be exceedingly high, as may systolic blood pressure, ventilation, and respiratory rate. It is therefore essential to habituate children to the equipment and procedures. A child should be allowed to practice, in a playlike atmosphere, the use of mouthpiece, nose clip, and ergometer, and to handle the stethoscope and blood pressure cuff before the actual test is performed. When information is collected for research, one should consider the initial meeting an orientation session, and discard all data obtained in it. This is especially important in intervention studies, or other longitudinal protocols, when valid baseline information must be obtained.

Ethical Issues

Not all procedures that are used with adults are ethically justifiable for children, unless indicated for clinical diagnosis. This is true for such invasive techniques as the direct Fick or the dye dilution determination of cardiac output, muscle biopsy, or intraarterial measurement of blood pressure; the liberal use of radiographic or radioisotope-based measurements; the use of such pain-inducing procedures as electrical stimulation of muscle, or the insertion of a thermistor for measuring tympanic temperature; the exposure to such hostile environments as extreme cold, extreme heat and humidity, or hypoxic conditions; or the induction of hypohydration to levels that may compromise health. It is the contention of this author that, even if parents give their consent and the child volunteers to participate, such methods should not be employed. A challenging area of research is the development of alternative, ethically justifiable, methods. The use of the CO_2 rebreathing procedure to assess cardiac output is an example of such an endeavor. It is hoped that the development of the nuclear magnetic resonance (NMR) technique and refined electrophysiologic methods will obviate the need for muscle biopsies.

Special Child Populations

Exercise testing of some groups is particularly challenging. These include the preschoolers, the mentally retarded, and those with advanced motor disability. Preschoolers, especially those under 4 years, seldom have the motivation to exert intensely, nor the level of cooperation that is required for successful tests. As a result, few researchers have attempted to work with the preschool child (32–34). Similar problems have been encountered with the severely mentally retarded child, notably the trainable mentally retarded (35). The challenge in testing children with severe motor disability is the unsuitability of the commonly used ergometers. A cerebral palsied child with spastic diplegia, for example, who cannot dorsiflex his foot, may be able to pedal only part of a revolution on the cycle ergometer. The same child may be able, however, to complete a full pedal revolution when cycling in the semiprone position. The author's laboratory is currently attempting to modify an ergometer so that it can be used at a semiprone position.

A special, so far unresolved, problem is that of a child with markedly atrophic or dystrophic muscles. Patients with advanced stages of progressive muscular dystrophy or of rheumatoid arthritis, for example, produce extremely low peak mechanical power. Some cannot reach even 5 watts (author's data), compared with 250 watts in a healthy 10 year old boy. Such low loads cannot be produced or registered by existing ergometers, even at "zero resistance." The Spinal Cord Unit at the Chedoke-McMaster Hospitals, together with the author's laboratory, is currently attempting the construction of a wheelchair ergometer that can produce such low loads.

STUDYING THE EFFECTS OF TRAINING

A major challenge in the study of training in children and adolescents is posed by the confounding effects of growth and maturation. Various physiologic changes that are induced by training occur also during growth per se. These include, among others, a reduction in submaximal heart rate (18), ventilation (22), respiratory rate (22), and oxygen uptake (23); and an increase in maximal muscle (36) and blood (22) lactate concentration, body fluid acidity (37), peak anaerobic power (38), muscle strength (39), muscle endurance (40), and velocity of movement (41).

A case in point is the metabolic cost of walking and running. This function, which is assessed by submaximal oxygen uptake, can decrease with aerobic-type training (e.g. long distance running at intensities that raise heart rate to 170–180 beat/minute) by as much as 10 ml/kg/minute (42). Growth per se is accompanied by a reduction in the same function of some 5 ml/kg/minute during the first 5 years of the second decade (18,23,43). The need to include a control group in any training-intervention study is thus obvious. For a review of the considerations regarding longitudinal design in training studies see Rutenfranz (44). An alternative approach is a mixed longitudinal cross-sectional design, in which training and growth effects can be separated (45).

When the assignment of subjects to experimental and control groups cannot be done randomly the controls must be chosen carefully. Because stages of maturation among adolescents of any given age vary widely, matching of groups must be based not on chronological age but rather on developmental age. Other variables to be matched include body size and composition, and the baseline level of fitness.

Another issue, yet unresolved, is how to equate the training stimulus across ages. If one is to compare, for example, the effects of a running program on prepubescents and pubescents, one must not use identical regimens in both groups. A regimen that is suitable for the prepubescent may be below the training threshold of the more mature individual. A possible approach for equating the intensity of training is the use of such indices as % maximal heart rate, % maximal aerobic power, or a certain rating of perceived exertion. It has yet to be determined which index is the most appropriate.

EXERCISE PRESCRIPTION FOR THE SICK CHILD

Children often use movement and physical play as a means of self-expression. Therefore, the need for sufficient exertion in a child—healthy or ill—is greater than in an adult. Healthy children seldom need an exercise prescription, unless they aspire to athletic excellence. In contrast, a child with an illness—actual or presumed—is often hypoactive when compared with his healthy peers (see Ref. 11 for a review). Such a child may require a specific exercise prescription to increase his fitness and to facilitate physical and psychosocial management and rehabilitation. An intelligent approach to a remedial exercise program ought to be problem-oriented. It must take into account the causes of hypoactivity in each patient and the specific physiologic and psychosocial objectives that are to be reached. The following are some examples.

Asthma. Asthmatic children often elect to be sedentary because of previous asthmatic attacks induced by exertion. Such children should be encouraged to pursue a swimming program. This is because of the well-documented low asthmogenicity of swimming, compared with land-based sports, such as running, cycling, or ball games (46–48). Among land-based activities short, intermittent ones seem preferable to those which are continuous in nature. These should be preceded by a warming up period of a few minutes (49,50).

The rationale for prescribing activity programs for asthmatics is an increase in general fitness, particularly in maximal aerobic power. Some reports (49,51,52), but not all (53,54), claim that training can also reduce the incidence and intensity of exercise-induced bronchoconstriction.

Childhood Obesity. The main physiologic objective in prescribing exercise for the obese is fat loss. The best activities, therefore, are those that require high energy expenditure, such as walking, jogging, swimming, or cycling. For the growing child or adolescent, weight loss per se should be deemphasized. Such an individual will often retain, or even increase, his body weight and still lose fat. This pattern is less likely in the obese adult. Obese children are often hypoactive (11,55). This may result from teasing by peers, social rejection, shame of exposing their "ugly" body, or loss of confidence in their physical prowess (56–58). Such individuals typically assume a vicious circle of hypoactivity, detraining, overweight, and further hypoactivity.

In choosing an exercise program (combined with dietary modification, whenever indicated) one must first instill confidence in the patient regarding his ability to exercise. Initial activities therefore need not be those with high calorie equivalence but those that the patient himself prefers. Only when some self-confidence has been built can the obese patient be encouraged to increase gradually the energy cost of his exercises. Even then, the set goals should be within his reach. Many obese patients will prefer not to join exercise programs which include their healthy peers. They would rather exert at home, or join classes with obese children or those with other disabilities. Swimming is the single best sport for the obese child: it requires high energy expenditure, the child is submerged such that his body is not exposed, and he can make good use of his high buoyancy.

Motor Disabilities. In diseases such as asthma or obesity, hypoactivity is incidental to the disease itself. In contrast, the low activity level and physical fitness of a child with muscular dystrophy, cerebral palsy, spina bifida, or juvenile rheumatoid arthritis is often a direct result of the pathophysiologic process. Thus, an exercise prescription for a child with motor disability must take into account the specific lesion, capitalizing on the residual motor abilities of the child. The functions to be improved include muscle strength, muscle endurance, and range of motion. An increase in maximal aerobic power should not be the main objective. As in other chronic diseases, the activity program for the child with motor disability must include a recreation component. Some patients, such as those with spina bifida or muscular dystrophy, are often obese. For them, exercise can be used also as a means of weight control. It should include prolonged tasks in which all, or most, body mass is moving.

REFERENCES

1. C. Thorén, Ed., *Pediatric Work Physiology,* Supplement No. 217, *Acta Paediatr. Scand.,* Stockholm (1971).

2. O. Bar-Or, Ed., *Pediatric Work Physiology,* Proceedings of the IVth International Symposium, Wingate Institute, Netanya, 1973.
3. J. Borms and M. Hebbelinck, Eds., *Children and Exercise,* Proceedings of the Vth International Symposium on Pediatric Work Physiology, *Acta Paed. Belg.*, Suppl. 28 (1974).
4. J. Borms and M. Hebbelinck, Eds., *Pediatric Work Physiology,* Proceedings of the VIth and VIII International Symposia, Karger, Basel, 1978.
5. H. Lavallée and R. J. Shephard, Eds., *Frontiers of Activity and Child Health,* Proceedings of the VIIth International Symposium of Pediatric Work Physiology, Pelican, Quebec, 1977.
6. K. Berg and B. O. Eriksson, Eds., *Children and Exercise IX,* University Park, Baltimore, 1980.
7. J. Ilmarinen and I. Valimaki, Eds., *Children and Sport,* Springer Verlag, Berlin, Heidelberg, 1984.
8. R. A. Binkhorst and W. H. M. Saris, Eds., *Proceedings of the XIth International Symposium of Pediatric Work Physiology,* Human Kinetics, Champaign, Ill., in press.
9. S. Godfrey, *Exercise Testing in Children,* Applications in Health and Disease, W. B. Saunders, Philadelphia, 1974.
10. R. J. Shephard, *Physical Activity and Growth,* Year Book Medical Publishers, Chicago, 1982.
11. O. Bar-Or, *Pediatric Sports Medicine For the Practitioner: From Physiologic Principles to Clinical Application,* Springer Verlag, New York, 1983.
12. N. J. Smith, Ed., *Sports Medicine: Health Care for Young Athletes,* Am. Acad. Pediatr., Evanston, Ill., 1983.
13. L. J. Micheli, Ed., *Pediatric and Adolescent Sports Medicine,* Little, Brown, Boston, 1984.
14. R. Boileau, Ed., *Advances in Pediatric Sport Sciences,* Vol. I, Human Kinetics, Champaign, Ill., 1984.
15. American Heart Association Council on Cardiovascular Disease in the Young, *Circulation,* **66,** 1377A (1982).
16. F. Klimt and G. B. Voigt, *Acta Paediatr. Scand.*, Suppl., **217,** 35 (1971).
17. M. Maček and J. Vávra, in K. Berg and B. O. Eriksson, Eds., *Children and Exercise IX,* University Park Press, Baltimore, 1980, p. 64.
18. J. S. Skinner, O. Bar-Or, V. Bergsteinová, C. W. Bell, D. Royer and E. R. Buskirk, *Acta Paediatr. Scand.*, Suppl., **217,** 24 (1971).
19. O. Bar-Or, *Symbioses,* **13,** 157 (1981).
20. L. Hermansen and S. Oseid, *Acta Paediatr. Scand.,* Suppl., **217,** 18 (1971).
21. B. Woynarowska, *Eur. J. Appl. Physiol.,* **43,** 19 (1980).
22. S. Robinson, *Int. Z. Angew. Physiol. Einschl. Arbeitsphysiol.,* **10,** 251 (1938).
23. P. O. Astrand, *Experimental Studies of Physical Working Capacity in Relation to Sex and Age,* Munksgaard, Copenhagen, 1952.
24. C. Thorén, in J. Borms and H. Hebbelinsk, Eds., *Pediatric Work Physiology,* Karger, Basel, 1978, p. 89.

25. M. R. H. Taylor and S. Godfrey, *Brit. Heart J.*, **34,** 930 (1972).
26. G. Cumming, *Am. J. Cardiol.*, **42,** 613 (1978).
27. R. Mocellin, in R. A. Binkhorst and W. H. M. Saris, Eds., *Pediatric Work Physiology XI,* Human Kinetics, Champaign, Ill., in press.
28. R. Sockolov, B. Irwin, R. H. Dressendorfer, and E. M. Bernauer, *Arch. Phys. Med.*, **58,** 195 (1977).
29. D. Ikkos and J. S. Hanson, *Circulation,* **22,** 583 (1960).
30. C. Thorén, P. Herin, and J. Vávra, *Acta Paed. Belg.*, **28,** Suppl., 132 (1974).
31. O. Inbar, Ed. D. Dissertation, Columbia University, 1978.
32. F. Klimt, *Acta Paediatr. Scand.*, Suppl., **217,** 32 (1971).
33. B. Mrzena and M. Maček, in J. Borms and H. Hebbelinsk, Eds., *Pediatric Work Physiology,* Karger, Basel, 1978, p. 29.
34. T. Yoshida, I. Ishiko and I. Muraoka, *Int. J. Sports Med.*, **1,** 91 (1980).
35. B. R. Londeree and L. E. Johnson, *Med. Sci. Sports,* **6,** 247 (1974).
36. B. O. Eriksson, J. Karlsson and B. Saltin, *Acta Paediat. Scand.*, Suppl., **217,** 154 (1971).
37. J. Matěkova, Z. Kopřivová, and Z. Placheta, in Z. Placheta, Ed., *Youth and Physical Activity,* J. E. Purkyne Univ., Brno, 1980, p. 191.
38. P. E. di Prampero and P. Cerretelli, *Ergonomics,* **12,** 51 (1969).
39. J. Vrijens, *Med. Sport* (Basel), **11,** 152 (1978).
40. O. Inbar and O. Bar-Or, *Med. Sci. Sports Exerc.*, in press.
41. E. Asmussen and K. R. Heeboll-Nielsen, *J. Appl. Physiol.*, **7,** 593 (1955).
42. J. Daniels and N. Oldridge, *Med. Sci. Sports,* **3,** 161 (1971).
43. J. D. MacDougall, P. D. Roche, O. Bar-Or and J. R. Moroz, *Int. J. Sports Med.*, **4,** 194 (1983).
44. J. Rutenfranz, *Med. Sci. Sports Exerc.*, in press.
45. J. Daniels, N. Oldridge, F. Nagle, and B. White, *Med. Sci. Sports,* **10,** 200 (1978).
46. K. D. Fitch and A. R. Morton, *Brit. Med. J.*, **4,** 577 (1971).
47. S. D. Anderson, Ph.D. Thesis, University of London, 1972.
48. O. Inbar, R. Dotan, R. A. Dlin, I. Neuman and O. Bar-Or, *Eur. J. Appl. Physiol.*, **44,** 43 (1980).
49. S. Oseid and K. Haaland, in B. Eriksson and B. Furberg, Eds., *Swimming Medicine IV,* Univeristy Park Press, Baltimore, 1978, p. 32.
50. R. Schnall, L. I. Landau, and P. D. Phelan, in S. Oseid and A. M. Edwards, Eds., *The Asthmatic Child in Play and Sport,* Pitman, Bath, 1983, p. 107.
51. J. M. Henriksen and T. Nielsen, *Acta Paediatr. Scand.*, **72,** 31 (1983).
52. E. Svenonius, R. Kautto, and M. Arborelius, Jr., *Acta Paediatr. Scand.*, **72,** 23 (1983).
53. K. D. Fitch, A. R. Morton and B. A. Blanksby, *Arch. Dis. Child.*, **51,** 190 (1976).
54. I. L. Swann and C. A. Hanson, in S. Oseid and A. M. Edwards, Eds., *The Asthmatic Child in Play and Sport,* Pitman, Bath, 1983, p. 318.

55. J. Mayer, in M. Winick, Ed., *Childhood Obesity,* Wiley, New York, 1975, p. 73.
56. H. Bruch, *Am. J. Dis. Child.,* **60,** 1082 (1940).
57. B. A. Bullen, L. F. Monello, H. Cohen, and J. Mayer, *Am. J. Clin. Nutr.,* **12,** 1 (1963).
58. N. Allon, *Am. J. Clin. Nutr.,* **32,** 470 (1979).

8

Effect of Exercise and Diet on Lipids and Cardiovascular Disease

EDWARD W. D. COLT, M.D.
and SAMI HASHIM, M.D.

Department of Medicine, St. Luke's-Roosevelt Hospital Center, New York, New York

Coronary heart disease (CHD) is responsible for 550,000 deaths in the United States each year—more than all forms of cancer put together. There are over 5.4 million Americans with symptomatic coronary disease, and a large number of others in whom the disorder is undiagnosed. Each year there are 1.5 million heart attacks. Coronary heart disease costs the country over $60 billion directly and indirectly. The disease reached its zenith in the 1960s, since when its incidence has fallen precipitously (1). Between 1968 and 1982, mortality from CHD has fallen by 32%, and that from stroke has fallen by 48% in the same period (2). Studies done on cardiovascular diseases, other than CHD, stroke in particular, suggest that they resemble CHD in their epidemiology and pathogenesis (3). In this chapter we shall use the term CHD to include myocardial infarction, angina pectoris, and sudden cardiac death. CHD serves as a useful endpoint for clinically diagnosing cardiovascular disease in large scale studies.

Lifestyle improvement seems to be the chief cause of the decrease in CHD mortality. It is difficult to separate out individual risk factors as each tends to affect the others. Surveys carried out since 1960 have shown a 29% decrease in smoking, a marked increase in the control of hypertension, a decrease in cholesterol consumption from 800 mg/day to < 500 mg/day, and a 40% decrease in the consumption of animal fat. In spite of the obvious overall increase in exercise in the last one or two decades, it has been stated that improvement in other risk factors would suffice to explain the decrease in cardiac deaths since 1970 (3).

Individuals who exercise most during their leisure are probably the ones most likely to stop smoking, eat a healthy diet, and have their blood pressure monitored. People who exercise regularly tend to come from the most highly educated sections of society; this group also tend to be less obese, smoke less, and have lower cholesterol levels than those who are less well educated. The highest death rate from CHD in the United States occurs at the lowest socioeconomic and educational levels (4–5). Even in the absence of other risk factor improvements, there is compelling evidence that exercise protects against atherosclerosis.

EFFECT OF EXERCISE ON LIPIDS AND CARDIOVASCULAR DISEASE

Epidemiological Studies

Many studies agree on the association between exercise and protection from heart disease. Only the landmark studies will be discussed in this chapter. The first to report this association was by Morris and coworkers in 1953 (7). They studied the occurrence of coronary heart disease in drivers and conductors of buses, trams, and trolleybuses, and also in postal workers. In all, the study included about 424,000 man-years of observation. The results showed that "men in physically active jobs have a lower incidence of coronary heart disease in middle age than have men in physically inactive jobs. More important, the disease is not so severe in physically active workers, tending to present first in them as angina pectoris and other relatively benign forms, and to have a smaller early case fatality and a lower early mortality rate."

The authors believed that physical activity might be the cause of the lower incidence of heart disease in the conductors than in the drivers. However they pointed out that the differences could also have been due to constitution and early experience, and that the men select the jobs for which they are best suited. Another factor could have been the different mental strains in driving and conducting.

Then there was the London Civil Service study (8) in which the leisure time exercise habits of middle aged civil servants were examined by questionnaire. Men who engaged in vigorous sports, kept fit, and the like during an initial survey in 1968–70 had an incidence of CHD in the next 8½ years somewhat less than half that of their colleagues who recorded no vigorous exercise. The CHD rates of men who took vigorous exercise were lower in both fatal and nonfatal clinical manifestations, though more so in fatal; throughout the age range studied, though more striking in later middle age and early old age; and in all other subgroups examined, including men with a family history of CHD, the obese, the short of stature, cigarette smokers, and men with severe hypertension, and subclinical angina, as well as those in favorable or neutral situations for CHD.

Once again from this study it was not possible to know whether exercise offered protection against heart disease or whether people with healthier hearts took more exercise.

Paffenbarger and coworkers (9) reported a 22 year follow-up of 3686 San Francisco longshoremen with particular regard to physical activity, and the well-known risk factors for CHD. The average energy output per 10 hour workday for the arbitrarily defined low energy workers was rated at 1066 kcal in excess of basal requirements, and for high energy workers at 1976 kcal. There was a 97% added risk of heart attack associated with the lower level of energy expenditure. There was also a 62% added risk of stroke associated with the lower level of energy expenditure, although this latter difference was not statistically significant. In parenthesis, it should be added that Salonen and coworkers also found that low physical activity was associated with an increased incidence of stroke (10). When men who actively loaded cargo were promoted to the less physically demanding job of crane operator, their risk of heart attack increased within a few months. This argued in favor of activity rather than genetic endowment as the cause of the protection from heart disease.

Paffenbarger and coworkers (11) studied 17,000 Harvard alumni by a very extensive questionnaire which went into all the details of the subject's lifestyle that could possibly have been related to CHD—namely, age, cigarette smoking, alcohol consumption, exercise habits, and so forth. They found that whatever group was studied, the people who exercised had less heart attack than those who were sedentary. As little as climbing five flights of stairs a day reduced the incidence of heart attacks by 25%. More vigorous exercises, such as squash or running, conferred greater protection than walking or golf for any given level of caloric expenditure. Individuals who had represented the college in a sport had no less incidence of myocardial infarction (MI) than those who had not been athletes in college—unless they continued to exercise. This argued strongly that it was the exercise itself rather than heredity (or constitution) which protected against heart disease, as did the fact that the protective effect of exercise lasted only about six months after exercise was discontinued. The maximum protective effect of exercise against myocardial infarction was reached at a caloric expenditure of 2000 calories/week, which is equivalent to jogging about 20 miles/week.

The latter is in striking contrast to the marked differences in incidence of heart disease between longshoremen who expended about 10,000 calories per week compared with those who expended 5000 calories per week. It may well be that there were other lifestyle differences which explain this disparity.

Shephard and coworkers (12) followed a group of 610 postcoronary patients for an average of 36.5 months. These patients had been enrolled in an exercise centered rehabilitation program. They found that exercise compliance had a favorable effect on prognosis. Relative to regular participants, the risk ratio for fatal and nonfatal reinfarctions was 23.6 times higher among those who complied poorly with a prescribed exercise program.

While exercise itself could be having a beneficial effect on prognosis, alternative explanations of the association include (a) an association between poor exercise compliance and an adverse attitude to health (reflected in such practices as continued cigarette smoking), and (b) an association between poor exercise compliance and disease severity. Critics of cardiac rehabilitation claim that those with the most severe disease comply least, and it is the severity of the disease rather than the poor compliance which is the cause of the recurrences. There is insufficient available data for this question to be resolved.

In spite of this impressive body of evidence, it is important to remember that sudden cardiac death occurs much more frequently during vigorous exercise than at rest—even in people who habitually exercise. In the latter group, sudden death occurs five times more frequently during vigorous exercise than at rest. In sedentary people, sudden cardiac death occurs 56 times more frequently during exercise than at rest (13). This statistic has immense clinical application among middle aged runners, a significant proportion of whom have underlying CHD. Some of these run while they are having symptoms in the mistaken belief that by continuing to run they can ward off the consequences of their condition. This sequence of events was dramatized by the sudden death while jogging, of the runner-writer Jim Fixx in July 1984. He had been running 70 miles a week for many years, and in the weeks prior to his death, had complained of chest pain, but had declined to consult a physician or have a stress test.

Animal Studies

However convincing epidemiological studies are, the evidence that they provide is circumstantial. Direct evidence that exercise prevents atherosclerosis is difficult to obtain in human beings. Kramsch and coworkers (14) looked at the effect of treadmill exercise on developing coronary artery disease in monkeys on an atherogenic diet. A training effect was demonstrated by low heart rates. The serum total cholesterol levels were very high but the same (statistically) in exercising and nonexercising monkeys (around 620 mg/dl). However, in the exercise conditioned group receiving the atherogenic diet, there was also a small but significant ($p < .01$)) increase in the HDL cholesterol content compared with the sedentary group on the same diet. Similarly the rise in total triglycerides was significantly smaller in the exercise group—mainly due to a reduction in LDL and VLDL triglyceride content. Ischemic electrocardiographic changes, angiographic signs of coronary artery narrowing, and sudden death were observed only in nonconditioned monkeys, in which post mortem examination revealed marked coronary atherosclerosis and stenoses.

In the sedentary monkeys, the atherogenic diet induced grossly visible coronary atherosclerosis. In contrast, coronary arteries of exercised monkeys had much less atheromatous involvement and considerably greater caliber, even at involved segments. The mean proportions of involvement of the coronary arteries were 60 ± 29% (left anterior descending), 52 ± 16% (left circumflex), and 46 ± 18% (right coronary) in sedentary monkeys, and 15 ± 11% (left anterior descending), 18 ± 8% (left circumflex), and 20 ± 5% (right coronary) in exercised animals. These differences were significant ($p < .01$).

Although the intimal lesions in sedentary monkeys were frequently fibrotic, lesions in exercised monkeys contained little if any collagen and consisted of lipid laden foam cells. In addition, the intimal thickening was less in exercised than in sedentary monkeys. Furthermore there was a significant increase in the size of the coronary artery lumina outlined by the internal elastica in conditioned monkeys as compared with both the internal elastic laminar lumina of sedentary animals on the atherogenic diet and those of the sedentary controls on a normal (nonatherogenic) diet.

The exercise group ran for 1 hour three times a week at a speed of 2.0–3.5 km/hour on a motorless treadmill with the exception of one monkey who ran very erratically and eventually did not exercise for more than 5 to 10 minutes per session. The proportions of involvement of the coronary arteries in this lazy monkey were intermediate between those of the exercising and sedentary monkeys. The level of exercise in the fully conditioned group was comparable to jogging in human beings.

In monkeys, exercise for as little as half an hour a week affords some protection against heart disease, and 3 hours a week affords even greater protection. Intuitively one might make similar predictions in humans, bearing in mind that the lifespan, and rate of evolution of atherosclerosis are different between the two species, and that therefore one might infer that the amount of exercise needed to protect against heart disease might have to be very different. Also the monkeys were consuming an even more atherogenic diet than is contained in a junk food diet, that is, hamburgers, frankfurters, eggs, ice cream, candies, cakes, and so forth.

MECHANISM OF PROTECTIVE EFFECT OF EXERCISE ON CHD

Exercise Mediated Changes in Lipids

The most striking change is the decrease in total and LDL cholesterol, and an increase in HDL cholesterol. Martin and coworkers (15) reported the total cholesterol levels of a group of elite runners with a mean age of 28 to be 175. Age matched good runners had a mean cholesterol of 185, while sedentary subjects had a cholesterol of 189. They were all eating a standard American diet. In these groups HDLs were 56, 52, and 49, respectively, while TGs were 74, 73, and 92, respectively. These authors also reported that total cholesterol increased with increasing age in both runners and sedentary subjects (from age 20 to 60). However whereas HDL increased with increasing age in runners, it decreased with increasing age in sedentary subjects.

There are a number of ways in which exercise could lower the blood levels of total and LDL cholesterol. Regular exercise causes an increase in plasma volume of as much as 20% (16). Thus a significant proportion of the lowering of serum cholesterol may be dilutional. There are no studies available comparing the total body cholesterol of exercisers and sedentary subjects. Simko and Kelley (17) reported that brisk walking causes a markedly increased hepatic secretion of bile and cholesterol, and presumably therefore increased transport of lipids from the periphery to the liver. Increased excretion of bile acids would diminish the total body cholesterol pool and lower the levels of total and LDL cholesterol.

There is a negative relation between HDL and the incidence of CHD (18–20). Regular exercise is associated with an increased level of HDL (21). Glomset has suggested that the transport of cholesterol from peripheral tissues to the liver, for subsequent catabolism and excretion, may be a function of HDL (22). Miller and Miller (19) have reported that total cholesterol pools of the body increase with decreasing plasma HDL concentrations but that total cholesterol pools are unrelated to plasma concentrations of total cholesterol.

How exercise increases HDL is not clear, but there is evidence that the increase is mediated by catecholamines. Physical training increases HDL in dogs, but in dogs receiving propranolol, HDL decreased despite physical training (23). Walker and coworkers (24) found that the HDL of male cardiac patients undergoing an exercise training program increased by 3.4% when they were put on beta blockers, whereas the HDL increased by 9.4% in the patients not on beta blockers.

Regular exercise is associated with a reduction in total triglycerides (TG) and VLDL (15). There is rather weak evidence linking these lipid fractions to CHD (25). The association between elevated levels of TG and CHD may be mediated by other associated risk factors, such as obesity, diabetes mellitus, and sedentariness, and there is a sizable negative correlation of triglyceride with HDL (26). Epstein and coworkers (27) have reported that there is an impaired fibrinolytic response to exercise in Type IV hyperlipoproteinemia; this would provide a direct link between atherosclerosis and raised plasma levels of TG or VLDL.

Exercise Mediated Reduction in Blood Pressure

Regular running causes a decrease in blood pressure in normotensive individuals (28–31). Many studies have shown that exercise programs lower blood pressure in hypertensive patients by as much as 20/18 mm Hg, and some of the reduction in blood pressure occurs independant of weight loss (32–44). Blood pressure is, of course, an important risk factor for CHD (45–65).

One of the ways in which exercise may lower blood pressure is by lowering adrenergic tone. This is suggested by the characteristically lower heart rate (66–71) and lower plasma renin activity (PRA) (72) in physically conditioned subjects. However the lowered PRA in resting athletes could also be attributed to plasma volume expansion. This lower adrenergic tone in trained subjects with a decreased sympathetic response to physical and psychological stress represents reduced risk for CHD (73).

Effect of Exercise on Plasma Volume

One of the causes of the decrease in blood pressure is the decrease in blood viscosity caused by running (72). This is presumably caused by the increase in plasma volume, but there is also a disproportionate decrease in the level of fibrinogen. The latter exerts a larger influence on plasma viscosity than globulin or albumin (72). For a given perfusion pressure and resistance vessel caliber, a decreased blood viscosity would decrease viscous resistance and increase blood flow. This effect would presumably mitigate the pressure gradient across a stenosed (coronary) artery, thereby maintaining perfusion.

In well-trained subjects, exercise increases the plasma volume acutely even in the face of marked dehydration. Colt and coworkers (74) found that despite a mean weight loss of 2.3% following a 10 mile run, there was a 2.6% increase in plasma volume in highly trained runners. Astrand and Saltin (75) found an 11% increase in plasma volume during an 85 km ski race that resulted in a 5.5% decrease in body weight. Convertino and coworkers (76) showed that over an 8 day interval a 10–15% increase in plasma volume was produced by bicycling for 2 hours/day. Few if any studies have been done on the effect of intense exercise on the plasma volume of untrained subjects, but clinically it is well known that exercise in the untrained rapidly results in all the manifestations of vascular collapse. The effect of acute exercise on trained patients with underlying CHD would be to reduce viscosity and resistance to flow in the stenosed vessels, thereby improving perfusion. The converse would be the case in untrained individuals with CHD, and the consequences could be disastrous.

Decrease in Body Weight and Adiposity

Training decreases body weight and adiposity in nonobese subjects (77), although it may cause weight gain in people suffering from hyperplastic obesity (78). Adiposity is a cardiac risk factor (79–85).

Reduction in Anxiety

Regular exercise reduces anxiety (86) and depression (87), both of which have been causally associated with CHD (88).

Protective Effects on Arterial Wall

There appear to be local effects of exercise on the arterial wall, which protect from atherosclerosis. Acid cholesteryl esterase was increased 20–30% above control levels in the aortas of rats on an 8 week, 1 hour/day swimming protocol (89). The authors speculated that this change could alter lipid accumulation in the blood vessel wall. Wolinsky earlier suggested that a reduced level of acid cholesteryl esterase might be a risk factor for coronary heart disease (90). The arbitrary separation of local effects on arterial walls from those of lipids may be artificial—sera from physically active individuals have been found to be less atherogenic than those of sedentary subjects in cultured human aortic smooth muscle cells (91).

Effects on Fibrinolysis and Fibrinogen

Exercise causes increased fibrinolysis (92), and regular training decreases the level of fibrinogen (72), both of which would have a protective effect against CHD (93–97).

Effects on Fasting Blood Sugar and Plasma Insulin Levels

Regular exercise reduces fasting blood sugar and plasma insulin levels in nonobese (98–101) and obese subjects (102). These changes are due to increased tissue sensitivity to insulin (103–106) mainly caused by the increase in concentration of insulin receptors (104,106). Increased levels of glucose (107–121) and insulin (116,122, 123) have been associated with CHD. Hyperglycemia is associated with nonenzymatic glycosylation of many proteins including collagen; glycosylated collagen traps LDL cholesterol even in the presence of the normal levels (of LDL cholesterol), thus providing a mechanism for the well-known propensity of diabetics to CHD (124).

General Health Consciousness

There can be little doubt that people who exercise regularly are particularly health conscious and more likely to make health promoting changes in all aspects of their lives. Although difficult to document, such an hypothesis accords well with clinical experience. Associations have been reported between educational level and improvement in activity, adiposity, diet, and the level of cholesterol (125,126).

EFFECT OF DIET ON LIPIDS AND CARDIOVASCULAR DISEASE

Thirty-three years have elapsed since Groen and associates (127) first demonstrated by means of a well-controlled study of 9 months duration in 60 normal volunteers, that substitution of vegetable for animal fats in the diet reduced the serum cholesterol. During the same year Kinnel and coworkers (128) reported that ingestion of diets containing relatively large amounts of vegetable fat consistently resulted in a significant fall in the level of serum cholesterol in human subjects. These observations have been amply confirmed. It is now clear that serum levels of cholesterol and LDL can be changed significantly when the pattern of fatty acids in the diet is rearranged. When the glycerides of dietary fats contain predominantly saturated long chain fatty acids (animal fats and coconut oil) concentrations of serum cholesterol and LDL tend to rise. When such dietary glycerides contain an appreciable proportion of polyunsaturated omega-6 fatty acids (most vegetable fats, essential or nonessential), serum cholesterol and LDL tend to decrease. The degree of change in serum lipids seems to depend on the magnitude of change in the fatty acid composition of the diet. It soon became apparent that it was not practicable, and perhaps was even harmful, to achieve a total switch in fat intake from animal to sunflower, sesame, and cotton seed oil. Olive oil, a delectable vegetable fat, was considered neutral to mildly hypocholesterolemic. There has been a tremendous increase in the consumption of vegetable oils and the margarines derived from them. Conversely, the consumption of animal fats (contained in red meat and dairy products) has dropped. Further studies have showed that one need not ''bathe'' in oils to lower cholesterol and that a diet with admixed triglycerides (10% saturated, 10% polyunsaturated; 10% monounsaturated) providing 30% of calories from fat and at the same time low in cholesterol (<250 mg/day) was palatable and efficacious in lowering serum cholesterol and LDL. Such a diet, or a modification thereof, formed the basis for most of the clinical trials involving the effect of diet on serum lipids and mortality from CHD.

Recent studies have shown that some vegetable fibers may reduce the level of serum cholesterol and LDL. Reports indicate that in several animal species atherosclerosis may have been reduced by feeding vegetable fibers derived from oat bran, wheat straw, rice bran, or alfalfa (129). In man, the cholesterol lowering seems to be induced by such fibers as pectin and gums. Moreover the vegetable fibers and vegetable derived proteins appear to enhance the cholesterol lowering effect of fat modified diets in man (130).

There are now many studies showing the association between diet, lipids, and cardiovascular disease. A report from the World Health Organization showed a correlation coefficient of +0.47 between total fat consumption and mortality from CHD in eighteen countries (131). There was a still closer correlation ($r = +.75$) between CHD mortality and the consumption of dairy fats in 22 countries (132).

The Zutphen study (Holland) reported recently (133) suggests that fish consumption is an independent negative risk factor for CHD. An inverse dose-response relation was found between fish consumption in 1960 and death from CHD during 20 years of follow-up of 852 men. Mortality from CHD was more than 50% lower among those who consumed 30 g of fish per day than among those who did not eat fish. These results are reminiscent of earlier studies indicating a low death rate from CHD among other communities with much higher average fish consumption, such as the Greenland Eskimos (400 g per day) (134), and the Japanese 100 g per day (135,136). Fish fat contains large quantities of long chain highly polyunsaturated omega-3 fatty acids, which have been found to be hypolipidemic in small scale metabolic studies (137,138). However in the Zutphen study, it was deemed unlikely that the inverse relation between fish consumption and CHD could be explained by changes in lipid and lipoprotein metabolism. Thus the mechanism whereby a modest fish intake protects against CHD remains unknown.

The seven country study (139) which started in 1957 was carried out in five European countries—Italy, Yugoslavia, Greece, Netherlands, and Finland—and in the United States and Japan. A close correlation ($r = .84$) was found between the nutritional intake of saturated fats and the incidence of CHD. As the levels of serum cholesterol were found to be highly correlated with the intake of saturated fat ($r = .89$) and with CHD ($r = .84$) (140), it seemed probable that the effect of saturated fat on CHD was mediated through serum cholesterol. This is the basis of the lipid hypothesis; namely, that dietary cholesterol and saturated fat raise the levels of serum cholesterol, which in turn promotes atherogenesis followed by thrombosis with resultant arterial occlusion.

One of the first trials of the effect of dietary intervention on the incidence of CHD was the Finnish Mental Hospital Study (141,142). The trial took place in two chronic mental hospitals. It started in 1959 when in one of the hospitals, the diet was changed so that the dairy fats present in the original diet were almost completely replaced by vegetable oils, mainly soybean oil; the other hospital was kept as the control, without any dietary change. In 1965 the diets in the two hospitals were reversed and continued until 1971.

Adherence to the diets was monitored by determining the fatty acid composition of needle biopsy samples taken from a large group of patients in each hospital. During the first 6 years the mean serum cholesterol level in Hospital N on the experimental diet was 216 mg% while that in Hospital K on the regular diet was 268. During the second 6 years when the diets were crossed over the mean serum cholesterol in Hospital N (now on the regular diet) was 267 mg% while that on Hospital K (now on the experimental diet) was 236 mg%. The coronary mortality in the hospitals consuming the experimental (low saturated fat) diet was about one half that in the hospitals consuming the regular diet. This difference was significant in Hospital N ($p < .02$), but not statistically significant in Hospital K ($p < .06$), which had a smaller number of patients. No differences were found in other causes of death including cerebrovascular disease and cancer.

The Oslo Heart Study reported a 47% reduction in the incidence of myocardial infarction in a prospective randomized 5 year trail of a diet low in saturated fat and cholesterol and smoking intervention in men at high risk of CHD (143). Serum cholesterol and tobacco consumption decreased 13% and 45% respectively in the intervention group. The findings of the Multiple

Risk Factor Intervention Trial (MRFIT) were inconclusive despite a 7.1% drop in mortality in the intervention group because the control group lowered their mortality 41% below anticipated rates (Multiple Risk Factor Intervention Trial Research Group)! The reason for the extraordinary decrease in mortality in the control group was the new public awareness of risk factors and CHD, reinforced by the patients' doctors telling them at their frequent examinations that they were at high risk (144).

More recently, a large multicenter, randomized, double blind study tested the efficacy of cholesterol lowering in reducing risk of CHD in 3806 asymptomatic middle aged men with hypercholesterolemia (145). The treatment group received the bile acid sequestrant cholestyramine and the control group received a placebo for an average of 7.4 years. Both groups followed a moderate cholesterol lowering diet. The cholestyramine group experienced an average plasma LDL cholesterol reduction of 20.3%, which was a 12.5% greater reduction than that in the controls. The cholestyramine group experienced a 19% reduction in risk of CHD ($p < .05$). In a sense the results were anticlimactic, given what was already believed regarding the effect of cholesterol on atherosclerosis. However, the study was so flawlessly designed that the conclusion that serum LDL cholesterol plays a causal role in CHD appears indisputable. It seems equally indisputable that lowering serum LDL cholesterol (and total cholesterol) reduces the risk of CHD.

There are reports of dietary induced atherosclerosis in many species, including dogs (146), ducks (147), geese (147,148), swine (149), rabbits (150–153), chickens (154), and monkeys (14). Regression of atherosclerotic lesions has been reported in several species, including chickens, dogs, pigeons, and monkeys (155–157). In animals as well as in man, high cholesterol diets raise the serum levels of total and LDL cholesterol. For example in Macaca Fascicularis monkeys fed Purina Monkey Chow with 0.1% cholesterol and 10% butter (by weight), total and LDL cholesterol increased by about 600%, total and LDL triglyceride increased by about 300%, and HDL cholesterol decreased insignificantly (14).

MECHANISM OF PROTECTIVE EFFECT OF DIET ON CHD

Effect of Diet on Lipids

Epidemiological studies have shown a high correlation (r = .84) between the intake of saturated fat and CHD. Also serum cholesterol levels were highly correlated (r = .89) with saturated fat intake and CHD (r = .81) (140). There is a large amount of other evidence, which has been referred to earlier, that the levels of total and LDL cholesterol are a major risk factor for CHD presumably by a direct effect on the arterial wall.

The benefit of fat modified diets on morbidity and mortality from CHD appears to be related to its lowering effect on serum cholesterol and LDL. The mechanism whereby fat modified diets reduce the levels of serum cholesterol and LDL still is not clear (158). An increase in the intake of polyunsaturated fat is associated with enhanced bile acid and sterol excretion (159,160). The LDL receptor hypothesis promulgated by Brown and Goldstein (161) has been proposed as a mechanism whereby fat modified diets influence the serum levels of cholesterol and LDL. For example, a high intake of dietary cholesterol and saturated fats makes cholesterol accumulate in the liver cells, thereby suppressing the manufacture of LDL receptors. When animals are fed diets high in cholesterol and saturated fat, their synthesis of receptors in the liver is suppressed by 90%, resulting in a buildup of LDL in the blood. In contrast, in animals maintained on low fat diets the number of LDL receptors is high and the animals degrade injected LDL rapidly (161). The concept that LDL receptor deficiency is not only genetically determined, as in familial hypercholesterolemia, but is also acquired, may offer a new insight into the mechanism of diet-induced changes in serum cholesterol and LDL.

As long ago as 1951 Barr and coworkers (18) reported that HDL levels were lower in subjects with coronary disease than in normal subjects. In contrast there is an association between high levels of HDL and protection from heart disease, as previously mentioned. Cholesterol exists within the body in esterified and unesterified forms, but only the latter can exchange readily between plasma lipoproteins and tissue (22). The activity of the cholesterol esterifying enzyme, lecithin cholesterol acyltransferase (LCAT), has been shown to promote the transfer of cholesterol from erythrocytes to plasma by shifting the equilibrium towards esterified cholesterol (162). This process is accelerated by HDL (163), the unesterified portion of which is the preferred substrate for LCAT. Miller and Miller (19) have postulated a role for HDL in clearing tissue of cholesterol, as they have found an inverse relationship between plasma HDL levels and the size of the body cholesterol pool. In apparent confirmation of this, others have reported an inverse association between plasma levels of total and LDL cholesterol on the one hand versus HDL on the other (162–165). True as this may be within population groups that probably eat similar diets and are in other ways homogeneous, it is not true in cross-cultural studies. For example in a survey comparing lipid levels among boys in 16 countries, the correlation coefficient between the mean levels of total cholesterol and HDL for all individuals grouped into rural and urban areas was very high ($r = .90$, $p < .001$) (166). Also the Tarahumara Indians, among whom CHD is unknown, have mean levels of HDL that are extremely low (31 mg/dl) and might be considered predictive of CHD were they found in American subjects. The mean levels of total cholesterol in the Tarahumara were 125 mg% (167). One might therefore anticipate that the ratio HDL/total cholesterol or HDL/LDL cholesterol would be a better predictor of CHD than HDL alone or total cholesterol or HDL cholesterol, and this has been found (26). Although the ratio HDL/total cholesterol (or HDL/LDL) is a good predictor of CHD within a given population, such as that of Framingham, Massachussetts, there is no evidence to suggest that it is a useful predictor of CHD mortality in undeveloped countries where the diet contains much less saturated fat and the mean serum cholesterol is correspondingly lower. In the United States at the present time where various individuals and health conscious groups are making major dietary changes, the predictive power of this ratio may become less than heretofore when the diet was perhaps more uniform.

In 1977 the CHD mortality in men aged from 35 to 74 ranged from a maximum of 875 per 100,000 in Finland to a minimum of 100 in Japan. The death rate in the United States was high at 675 per 100,000. Since 1969 the United States has experienced a decrease of 200 CHD deaths per 100,000 (30%), the greatest decrease of any country in the world (168). During the same time interval, there has been an increase in the death rate from CHD in men in a number of countries, the greatest increase being in Bulgaria and Poland (168). In 1977 the CHD mortality for women ranged from a maximum of 360 per 100,000 in Northern Ireland to a minimum of 50 in Japan. In the United States the comparable figure was 264. As with men, there has been an impressive drop of 100 per 100,000 (38%) in CHD mortality among women in the United States (168). However during this time, CHD mortality in women has also increased in several other countries, the most striking increases being in Poland, Italy, and Rumania (168). These increases may represent "westernization" of dietary habits.

The mean level of serum cholesterol in the United States dropped from 225 mg% in 1952 to 205 mg%, 20 years later (169). During the same time the level of cholesterol describing the upper quintile of the population dropped from 265 mg% to 240 mg%—the data being derived from different populations. In the last two decades (1964–1984), it has been estimated that there has been a decrease of approximately 5% in the mean level of serum cholesterol of the population of the United States, adjusting for differences in methodology which may account for 3 to 5% of the apparent decrease (169).

Among the Tarahumara, with a mean level of plasma cholesterol of 125 mg%, CHD is unknown (167). In Japan the mean level of plasma cholesterol is 165 mg%, and the annual CHD mortality is 50 per 100,000 (168). Presumably the threshold below which CHD does not develop lies somewhere between plasma levels of cholesterol of 125 and 165 mg%, which should thus be the theoretical objective of our population. Blackburn and coworkers have suggested an ideal mean serum cholesterol of 160 +/−25 mg% for the population in general, with a feasible mean of 190 +/− 30 mg%, and a "present" (1979) mean of 210 mg%

(170). It has been repeatedly claimed, particularly by clinicians and cardiologists, that cholesterol levels cannot be lowered significantly by dietary measures because the appropriate food would be unpalatable. The marked decline in CHD mortality in the last two decades, which has accompanied the reduction of fat consumption, shows that dietary improvements are possible. There is no reason why further improvements will not follow if the trend towards decrease in fat consumption continues, as it surely will if Chinese, Japanese, and Mediterranean cuisine replace the high fat diet that is part of the northern European heritage of the industrialized world.

There is conflicting evidence that VLDL and triglycerides are a risk factor for CHD (84 171–183). However, the most recent view is that VLDL is not an independent risk factor but rather reflects changes in HDL with which there is an inverse association. Also VLDL may be elevated in diabetes mellitus, both clinical and subclinical, in which it is known that there is an increased risk of CHD (124).

Effects of Diet on Coronary Risk Factors

These effects will reduce CHD (largely) independent of lipoproteins.

Blood Pressure. Several short-term intervention studies have shown that lowering the quantity of saturated fat and increasing the P/S ratio in the diet cause decreases in blood pressure ranging from 8/5 to 13/7 mmHg (184–190). Polyunsaturated fats are the precursors of vasodilator and saluretic prostaglandins and this may well be how these dietary changes lower blood pressure (191).

In 1928 Addison suggested that the high prevalence of hypertension in North America was due to a high sodium, low potassium diet (192). Subsequently population studies have reported relationships between blood pressure and dietary sodium/potassium ratios (193–201). Intervention studies show that potassium supplements may lower blood pressure (particularly in subjects with essential hypertension) by as much as 9/6 mm Hg (185). Skrabel and coworkers (202) hypothesized that the beneficial effects by which a high potassium diet may improve blood pressure are 1. direct saluretic effect, 2. increased sensitivity of baroreceptor responses, 3. prevention of increased catecholamine response which follows sodium restriction, 4. improved patient compliance with low salt diet because salty foods are replaced by fruit and vegetables or salt substitutes.

It is interesting that diets low in saturated fats, with low sodium/potassium ratios and high P/S ratios are all found in the high fiber, low fat diet, suggesting perhaps that man has evolved to be a vegetarian. Any departure puts him at the mercy of foods with which he is not equipped to cope.

Sodium has of course long been known to be associated with increased blood pressure both in individuals and populations, but it is not appropriate to treat this important topic here.

Body Weight. High fiber, low fat diets promote weight loss (203) for reasons that have yet to be clearly defined—possibly because satiety is reached after the ingestion of a lower amount of calories than is contained in a high fat diet. The addition of guar gum to a low energy liquid meal significantly increases the viscosity of the meal and reduces the rate at which it leaves the stomach (204). Dietary fiber has been shown to inhibit cholesterol absorption directly (205). Thus a high fiber diet positively influences important coronary risk factors.

Health Consciousness. Health conscious people are more likely to eat what they perceive to be healthy diets. There can be little doubt that once a person has focused on one aspect of health, he or she is more likely to turn to other healthful habits, such as regular exercise, monitoring blood pressure, regulating the intake of salt, alcohol, and caffeine, cutting down on cigarette smoking, and so forth. As one might expect from behavior that can be learned, healthy interventions (of all kinds) have been made more frequently by people of higher education and income levels (5). Furthermore the incidence of CHD is less in more educated people than in less educated people (4).

REFERENCES

1. R. I. Levy, *Am. J. Cardiol.,* 1C. (Aug. 27, 1984).
2. M. Feinleib, *Am. J. Cardiol.,* **54,** 2C (1984).
3. R. I. Levy, *Am. J. Cardiol.,* 7C (Aug. 27, 1984).
4. L. E. Hinkle, Jr., L. H. Whitney, E. W. Lehman, et al., *Science,* **161,** 238 (1968).
5. J. Stamler, *Am. J. Cardiol.,* **47,** 772 (1981).
6. W. J. Walker, *New Engl. J. Med.,* 308, **11,** 649 (1983).
7. J. N. Morris, J. A. Heady, P. A. B. Raffle, C. G. Roberts, and J. W. Parks, *Lancet,* **2,** 1053, 1110 (1953).
8. J. N. Morris, S. P. W. Chave, C. Adam, et al., *Lancet,* **1,** 333 (1973).
9. R. S. Paffenbarger, Jr., R. J. Brand, R. I. Sholtz, and D. L. Jung, *Am. J. Epidemiol.,* **108,** 12 (1978).
10. J. T. Salonen, P. Puska, and J. Tuomilehto, *Am. J. Epidemiol.,* **115,** 526 (1982).
11. R. S. Paffenbarger, Jr., A. L. Wing, R. T. Hyde, *Am. J. Epidemiol.,* **108,** 161 (1978).
12. R. J. Shephard, P. Corey, and T. Kavanagh, *Med. Sci. Sports Exerc.,* **13,** 1 (1981).
13. D. S. Siscovick, N. S. Weiss, R. H. Fletcher, and T. Lasky, *N. Engl. J. Med.,* **311,** 874 (1984).
14. D. M. Kramsch, A. J. Aspen, B. M. Abramowitz, J. Kreimendahl, and W. B. Hood, *N. Engl. J. Med.,* **305,** 483 (1981).
15. R. P. Martin, W. L. Haskell, and P. D. Wood, *Ann. N.Y. Acad. Sci.,* **301,** 346 (1977).
16. J. Brotherhood, B. Brozovic, and L. G. C. Pugh, *Clin. Sci. Mol. Med.,* **48,** 138 (1975).
17. V. Simko and R. E. Kelley, *Athersclerosis,* **32,** 423 (1979).
18. D. P. Barr, E. M. Russ, and H. A. Eder, *Am. J. Med.,* **11,** 480 (1951).
19. A. J. Miller and N. E. Miller, *Lancet,* **1,** 16 (1975).
20. G. G. Rhoads, C. L. Gulbrandsen, and A. Kagan, *N. Engl. J. Med.,* **294,** 294 (1976).
21. P. D. Wood, W. L. Haskell, H. Klein, S. Lewis, M. P. Stern, and J. W. Farquhar, *Metabolism,* **25,** 1249 (1976).
22. J. A. Glomset, *J. Lipid Res.,* **9,** 155 (1968).
23. A. A. Bove, M. R. Lawlot, D. P. Thomas, J. Michele, and A. M. Paolone, Abstract, *Med. Sci. Sports Exerc.,* May, 124 (1983).
24. D. A. Walker, S. J. K. Lee, and R. M. McAllister, Abstract, *Med. Sci. Sports Exerc.,* May, 166 (1983).

25. R. Pelkonen, E. A. Nikkila, S. Koskinen, et al., *Brit. Med. J.* **2,** 1185 (1977).
26. T. Gordon, W. P. Castelli, M. C. Hjortland, W. B. Kannel, and T. R. Dawber, *Am. J. Med.,* **62,** 707 (1977).
27. S. E. Epstein, D. R. Rosing, P. Brakman, and D. R. Redwood, *Lancet,* **2,** 631 (1970).
28. K. H. Cooper, M. L. Pollack, R. P. Martin, et al., *J.A.M.A.,* **236,** 166 (1976).
29. P. D. Wood, W. L. Haskell, M. P. Stern, S. Lewis, and C. Perry, *Ann. N. Y. Acad. Sci.,* **301,** 748 (1977).
30. J. D. Cantwell, *J.A.M.A.,* **240,** 1409 (1978).
31. M. H. Criqui, I. Mebane, R. B. Wallace, et al., *Prev. Med.,* **11,** 391 (1982).
32. J. L. Boyer and F. W. Kasch, *J.A.M.A.,* **211,** 1668 (1970).
33. J. A. Bonnano and J. E. Lies, *Am. J. Cardiol.,* **33,** 760 (1974).
34. G. Choquette and R. J. Ferguson, *Can. Med. Assoc. J.,* **108,** 699 (1973).
35. M. Krotkiewski, K. Mandroukas, L. Sjostrom, et al. *Metabolism,* **28,** 650 (1979).
36. O. Roman, A. L. Camuzzi, E. Villalon, and C. Klenner, *Cardiology,* **67,** 230 (1981).
37. K. Pyorolo, R. Karava, S. Punsar, et al., in O. A. Larsen and R. O. Malmborg, Eds., *Coronary Heart Disease and Physical Fitness,* Munksgoard, Copenhagen, 1971.
38. J. F. DePlaen and J. M. Detry, *Acta Cardio.,* **35,** 179 (1980).
39. J. Ressl, J. Chrastek, and R. Handova, *Acta Cardiol.,* **32,** 121 (1977).
40. J. L. Rudd, and W. C. Day, *J. Am. Geri. Soc.,* **15,** 373 (1957).
41. R. Sannerstedt, H. Wasir, R. Hemming, and L. Werko, *Clin. Sci. Mol. Med.,* **45,** 1455 (1973).
42. J. Ilmarinen and P. S. Fardy, *Prev. Med.,* **6,** 416 (1977).
43. A. W. Sedgwick, J. R. Brotherhood, et al., *Brit. Med. J.,* **281,** 7 (1980).
44. J. Stamler, E. Farinaro, L. M. Mojonnier, et al., *J.A.M.A.,* **243,** 1819 (1980).
45. Pooling Project Group, *J. Chronic Dis.,* **31,** 201 (1978).
46. W. B. Kannel, *Aust. N.Z. J. Med.,* **6,** 373 (1976).
47. W. B. Kannel, *Aust. N.Z. J. Med.,* **6,** 410 (1976).
48. W. B. Kannel, *Am. J. Cardio.,* **37,** 269 (1976).
49. A. Keys, *Circulation,* Suppl. 1, 41 (1970).
50. T. L. Robertson, I. Kato, G. G. Rhoads, et al., *Am. J. Cardiol.,* **39,** 239 (1977).
51. H. C. McGill, J. Arias-Stella, L. M. Carbonell, et al., *Lab. Invest.,* **18,** 498 (1968).
52. A. J. Anderson, J. J. Barboriak, and A. A. Rimm, *Am. J. Epidemiol.,* **107,** 8 (1978).
53. J. C. Cassel, *Arch. Intern. Med.,* **128,** 883 (1971).
54. W. B. Kannel, *Med. Clin. North Am.,* **58,** 363 (1974).
55. T. R. Dawber, W. B. Kannel, N. Revotslei, et al., *Proc. R. Soc. Med.* **55,** 265 (1962).
56. H. M. Whyte, *Aust. N.Z. J. Med.,* **6,** 387 (1976).
57. A. Keys, C. Aravanis, H. Blackburn, et al., *Circulation,* **45,** 815 (1972).

58. G. Rose, P. J. S. Hamilton, H. Keen, et al., *Lancet,* **1,** 105 (1977).
59. O. Paul, M. H. Lepper, W. H. Phelan, et al., *Circulation,* **28,** 20 (1963).
60. R. S. Paffenbarger, R. J. Brand, R. I. Scholtz, et al., *Am J. Epidemiol.,* **108,** 12 (1978).
61. A. Keys, H. L. Taylor, H. Blackburn, et al., *Arch. Intern. Med.,* **128,** 201 (1971).
62. S. W. Rabkin, F. A. L. Mathewson, and P. H. Hsu, *Am. J. Cardiol.,* **39,** 452 (1977).
63. W. B. Kannel, T. Gordon, M. J. Schwartz, *Am. J. Cardiol.,* **27,** 335 (1971).
64. J. W. Gofman, W. Young, R. Tandy, *Circulation,* **34,** 679 (1966).
65. H. A. Tryoler, S. Heyden, A. Bartel, et al., *Arch. Intern. Med.,* **128,** 907 (1971).
66. P. O. Astrand, *Prog. Cardiovasc. Dis.,* **19,** 51 (1976).
67. B. Ekblom and L. Hermanson, *J. Appl. Physiol.,* **25,** 619, (1968).
68. B. Ekblom, P. O. Astrand, B. Saltin, J. Stenberg, and B. Wallstrom, *J. Appl. Physiol.,* **24,** 518 (1968).
69. L. B. Rowell, *Physiol. Rev.,* **54,** 75 (1971).
70. J. Scheuer and C. M. Tipton, *Ann. Rev. Physiol.,* **39,** 221 (1977).
71. R. D. Gordon, O. Kuchel, G. E. Liddle, D. P. Island, *J. Clin. Invest.,* **46,** 599 (1967).
72. R. L. Letcher, T. G. Pickering, S. Chien, J. H. Laragh, *Clin. Cardiol.,* **4,** 172 (1981).
73. C. H. Folkins and E. A. Amsterdam, ''Control and Modification of Stress Emotions through Chronic Exercise,'' in E. A. Amsterdam, J. H. Wilmore, A. N. DeMaria, Eds., *Exericse in Cardiovascular Health and Disease.* Yorke Medical, New York, 1977.
74. E. W. D. Colt, J. Wang, and R. N. Pierson, *J. Appl. Physiol.,* **45,** 999 (1978).
75. P. O. Astrand and B. Saltin, *J. Appl. Physiol.,* **19,** 829 (1964).
76. V. A. Convertino, J. E. Greenleaf, and E. M. Bernauer, *Physiologist,* **20,** 18 (1977).
77. P. Bjorntorp, G. Holm, B. Jacobsson, et al., *Metabolism,* **26,** 19 (1977).
78. M. Krotkiewski, K. Mandroukas, L. Sjostrom, L. Sullivan, H. Wetterquist, and P. Bjorntorp, *Metabolism,* **28,** 650 (1979).
79. Pooling Project Group, *J. Chronic Dis.,* **31,** 201 (1978).
80. W. B. Kannel, *Am. J. Cardiol.,* **37,** 269 (1976).
81. T. Zeiner-Henrikson, *J. Chronic Dis.,* **29,** 15-33 (1976).
82. D. Kozarevic, B. Pirc, T. R. Dawber, et al., *J. Cronic Dis.,* **29,** 405 and *Am. J. Epidemiol.,* **104,** 133 (1976).
83. S. W. Rabkin, F. A. L. Mathewson, and P. H. Hsu, *Am. J. Cardiol.,* **39,** 452 (1977).
84. T. Gordon, W. P. Castelli, M. C. Hjortland, et al., *Ann. Intern. Med.,* **87,** 393 (1977).
85. M. M. Gertler, P. D. White, L. D. Cady, et al., *Am. J. Med. Sci.,* **248,** 377 (1964).
86. W. P. Morgan, ''Influence of Acute Physical Activity on State Anxiety.'' *Proceedings of the National College Physical Education Association for men,* 1973, pp. 113-121.

87. J. H. Greist, M. H. Klein, R. R. Eischen, J. Faris, A. S. Gurman, and W. P. Morgan, *Comp. Psychiatry,* **20,** 41 (1979).
88. C. D. Jenkins, *N. Engl. J. Med.,* **294,** 987, 1033 (1976).
89. H. Wolinsky, S. Goldfisher, D. Katz, R. Markle, L. Gidez, S. Wassertheil-Smoller and B. Coltoff-Schiller, *Circ. Res.,* **45,** 546 (1979).
90. H. Wolinsky, *Ann. N.Y. Acad. Sci.,* **275,** 238 (1976).
91. M. Tammi, T. Ronnemaa, T. Vihaersaari, H. Saarni, A. Lehtonen, and J. Viikari, *Med. Biol.,* **57,** 118 (1979).
92. R. J. Cohen, S. E. Epstein, L. S. Cohen, and L. H. Dennis, *Lancet,* **2,** 1264 (1968).
93. T. W. Meade, R. Chakrabarti, and W. R. S. North, *Adv. Exp. Med. Biol.,* **82,** 219 (1977).
94. R. Chakrabarti, E. D. Hocking, G. R. Fearnley, et al., *Lancet,* **1,** 987 (1968).
95. N. A. Marsh and N. G. Shaper, *Adv. Exp. Med. Biol.,* **82,** 540 (1977).
96. D. P. Burkitt and H. C. Trowell, *Refined Carbohydrate Foods and Disease,* Academic, London, 1975, pp. 195–226.
97. H. C. Kwaan, *Adv. Exp. Med. Biol.,* **104,** 295 (1978).
98. P. C. Davidson, S. R. Shane, and M. J. Albrink, *Circulation,* **33,** 7 (1966).
99. P. Bjorntorp, M. Fahlen, G. Grimby, A. Gustafson, J. Holm, P. Renstrom, and T. Schersten, *Metabolism,* **21,** 1037 (1972).
100. P. Bjorntorp, P. Berchtold, G. Grimby, B. Lindhokm, H. Sanne, G. Tibblin, and L. Wilhelmsen, *Acta Med. Scand.,* **192,** 439 (1972).
101. D. Streja and D. Mymin, *J.A.M.A.,* **242,** 2190 (1979).
102. P. Bjorntorp, *Clin. Endocr. Metab.,* **5** 431 (1976).
103. D. Lohmann, F. Liebold, W. Heilmann, H. Senger, and A. Pohl, *Metabolism,* **27,** 521 (1978).
104. V. Koivisto, V. Soman, P. Conrad, R. Hendler, E. Nadel, and P. Felig, *J. Clin. Invest.,* **64,** 1011 (1979).
105. J. LeBlanc, A. Nadeau, M. Boylay, and S. Rousseau-Migneron, *J. Appl. Physiol.,* **46,** 235 (1979).
106. V. R. Soman, V. A. Koivisto, D. Deibert, P. Felig, and R. A. De Fronzo, *N. Engl. J. Med.,* **301,** 1200 (1979).
107. Pooling Project Group, *J. Chronic. Dis.,* **31,** 201 (1978).
108. W. B. Kannel, *Am. J. Cardiol.,* **37,** 269 (1976).
109. F. H. Epstein, *Bull. N.Y. Acad. Med.,* **44,** 916 (1968).
110. H. Keen, *Postgrad. Med. J.,* **52,** 445 (1976).
111. F. H. Epstein and B. Chir, *Triangle,* **12,** 3 (1973).
112. H. Falsetti, D. Schnatz, D. Greene, et al. *Chest,* **58,** 111 (1970).
113. F. H. Epstein, L. D. Ostrander, B. C. Johnson, et al., *Ann. Intern. Med.,* **62,** 1170 (1965).
114. L. D. Ostrander, T. Francis, N. S. Hayner, et al., *Ann. Intern. Med.,* **62,** 1188 (1965).
115. H. Keen, G. Rose, D. A. Pyke et al. *Lancet,* **2,** 505 (1965).

116. R. W. Stout, *Atherosclerosis,* **27,** 1 (1977).

117. C. F. Howard *Adv. Exp. Med. Biol.,* **60,** 13 (1975).

118. K. M. West, *Epidemiology of Diabetes and its Vascular Lesions,* Elsevier, New York, 1978.

119. M. Brownlee and G. F. Cahill, *Atherosclerosis Rev.,* **4,** 29 (1979).

120. J. W. Anderson, *Am. J. Clin. Nutr.,* **28,** 273 (1975).

121. E. G. Lufkin, F. N. Fass, W. M. O'Fallon, et al., *Metabolism,* **28,** 63 (1979).

122. R. W. Stout, *Lancet,* **2,** 702 (1968).

123. R. W. Stout, *Atherosclerosis,* **27,** 271 (1977).

124. A. Cerami, H. Vlassara, M. Brownlee, ''Protein Glycosylation in Pathogenesis of Atherogenesis, in press.

125. J. Stamler, *Am. J. Cardio.,* **47,** 722 (1981).

126. L. E. Hinkle Jr., L. H. Whitney, E. W. Lehman, et al. *Science,* **161,** 238 (1968).

127. J. Groen, B. K. Tjiong, C. E. Kaminga, and A. F. Willebrands, *Voeding,* **13,** 556 (1952).

128. L. W. Kinsell, J. W. Partridge, L. A. Boling, S. Margen, and G. D. Michaels, *J. Clin. Endocrinol.,* **12,** 909 (1952).

129. R. M. Kay and A. S. Truswell, ''Dietary Fiber: Effects in Plasma and Biliary Lipids, in *Medical Aspects of Dietary Fiber,* G. A. Spiller and R. M. Kay, Eds, Plenum, New York, 1980.

130. B. Lewis, F. Hammett, M. B. Katan, R. M. Kay, I. Merka, A. Noble, N. E. Miller, and A. V. Swan, *Lancet,* **2,** 1310 (1981).

131. World Health Organization, *World Health Statistics Annual 1973,* Vol. I; World Health Organization, Geneva, 1976.

132. OECD/OCDE, *Food Consumption Statistics, 1955–1973,* Paris, 1975.

133. D. Kromhout, E. B. Bosschieter, and C. D. L. Coulander, *New Engl. J. Med.,* **312,** 1205 (1985).

134. H. O. Bang, J. Dyeberg, and H. M. Sinclair, *Am. J. Clin. Nutr.,* **33,** 2657 (1980).

135. A. Keys, Seven Countries: A Multivariate Analysis of Death and Coronary Heart Disease, Harvard University Press, Cambridge, Mass; 1980.

136. Y. Kagawa, M. Nishizawa, M. Suzuki, et al., *J. Nutr. Sci. Vitaminol. (Tokyo),* **28,** 441 (1982).

137. E. H. Ahrens, Jr., W. Insull, Jr., J. Hirsch, W. Stoffel, N. L. Peterson, J. W. F. Farquhar, T. Miller, and J. Thomasson, *Lancet,* **1,** 115 (1959).

138. B. E. Phillipson, D. W. Rothrock, W. E. Connor, Harris, and D. R. Illingworth, *New Engl. J. Med.,* **312,** 1210 (1985).

139. A. Keys, Ed., Circulation 41 (Suppl I): 1970, pp 1, 9, 162.

140. A. Keys, J. T. Anderson, and F. Grande, *Metabolism,* **14,** 747 (1965).

141. O. Turpeinen, M. Miettinen, M. J. Karvonen, P. Roine, M. Pekkarinen, E. J. Lehtuosos, P. Alvirta, *Am. J. Clin. Nutr.,* **21,** 255 (1968).

142. M. Miettinen, O. Turpeinen, M. J. Karvonen, R. Eluoso, and E. Paavilainen, *Lancet,* **2,** 835 (1972).

143. I. Hjerman, K. Veve Byre, I. Home, and P. Leren, *Lancet,* **2,** 1303 (1981).

144. Multiple Risk Factor Intervention Trial Research Group, *J.A.M.A.*, **248,** 1466 (1982).
145. Lipid Research Clinics Coronary Primary Prevention Trial, *J.A.M.A.*, **251,** 351 (1984).
146. F. F. McAllister, R. Bertsh, J. Jacobsen, II, and G. D'Alessio, *Arch. Surg.*, **80,** 54 (1960).
147. J. B. Wolffe, V. A. Digilio, A. D. Dale, et al., *Am. J. Heart J.*, **38,** 467 (1949).
148. J. B. Wolffe, A. S. Hyman, M. B. Plungian, A. D. Dale, G. F. McGinnis, and M. B. Walkow, *J. Gerontol.*, **7,** 13 (1952).
149. R. P. Link, W. M. Pedersoli, and A. H. Safanie, *Atherosclerosis,* **15,** 107 (1972).
150. A. L. Myasnikov, *Circulation,* **17,** 99 (1958).
151. S. D. Kobernick and T. Hashimoto, *Lab. Invest.*, **12,** 638 (1963).
152. S. D. Kobernick and G. Niwayama, *Am. J. Pathol.*, **36,** 393 (1960).
153. J. T. Prior and D. D. Ziegler, *Am. J. Pathol.*, **80,** 50 (1965).
154. H. S. Weiss, F. D. Brown, P. Griminger, and H. Fisher, *J. Atheroscler. Res.*, **6,** 407 (1966).
155. R. G. De Palma, C. A. Hubay, W. Insull, Jr, A. V. Robinson, and P. H. Hartman, *Surg. Gynecol. Obstet.*, **131,** 633 (1970).
156. A. S. Daoud, J. Jarmolych, K. Fritz, and J. Augustyn, *Circulation,* **20,** (Suppl. III), 92, (1974).
157. D. J. Farrar, H. D. Green, W. D. Wagner, and M. G. Bond, *Circulation,* **47,** 425 (1980).
158. R. L. Jacobson, O. D. Taunton, J. D. Morrisett, A. M. Gotto, Jr., *Circulation,* **42,** 447 (1978).
159. P. J. Nestel, N. Havenstein, H. M. Whyte, D. Phil, T. J. Scott, and I. J. Cook, *N. Engl. J. Med.*, **288,** 379 (1973).
160. J. M. Potter and P. J. Nestel, *Am. J. Clin. Nutr.*, **29,** 546 (1976).
161. M. S. Brown and J. L. Goldstein, *Scient. Am.*, **251,** 58 (1984).
162. G. J. Miller and N. E. Miller, *Lancet,* **1,** 16 (1975).
163. J. A. Glomset, *Am. J. Clin. Nutr.*, **23,** 1129 (1970).
164. A. V. Nichols, *Adv. Biol. Med. Phys.*, **11,** 109 (1967).
165. E. Nikkila, *Scand, J. Clin. Lab. Invest.*, **5**(Suppl. 8),1 (1953).
166. J. T. Knuiman, R. J. J. Hermus, and J. G. A. J. Haitvast, *Atherosclerosis,* **36,** 529 (1980).
167. W. E. Connor, M. T. Cerquieira, R. W. Connor, R. B. Wallace, R. Malinow, and H. R. Casdorph, *Am. J. Clin. Nutr.*, **31,** 1131 (1978).
168. Report of Inter-society Commission for Heart Disease Resources, *Circulation,* **70,** 155A (1984).
169. W. V. Brown, H. Ginsber, W. Karmally, *Am. J. Cardiol.*, **54,** 27C (1984).
170. H. Blackburn et al., *Prev. Med.*, **8,** 612 (1979).
171. R. Pelkonen, E. A. Nikkila, S. Koskinen, et al., *Brit. Med. J.*, **2,** 1185 (1977).
172. R. H. Rosenman, R. J. Brand, C. D. Jenkins, et al., *J.A.M.A.*, **233,** 872 (1975).
173. L. A. Carlson and L. E. Bottiger, *Lancet,* **1,** 865 (1972).

174. F. Martin and G. Warne, *Metabolism,* **24,** 1 (1975).

175. A. J. Anderson, J. J. Barboriak, and A. A. Rimm, *Am. J. Epidemiol.,* **107,** 8 (1978).

176. A. M. Gotto, G. A. Gorry, Thompson, Jr. et al., *Circulation,* **56,** 875 (1977).

177. P. F. Cohn, S. I. Gabbay, W. B. Weglicki, *Ann. Intern. Med.,* **84,** 241 (1976).

178. A. Bloch, R. E. Dinsmore, and R. S. Lees, *Lancet,* **1,** 928 (1976).

179. J. J. Barboriak, A. A. Rimon, A. J. Anderson, et al., *Am. Heart J.,* **87,** 716 (1974).

180. A. M. Gotto, *Atherosclerosis Rev.,* **4,** 17 (1979).

181. M. Tzagournis, *Am. J. Clin. Nutr.,* **31,** 1437 (1978).

182. T. Gordon, W. P. Castelli, M. C. Hjorrland, et al., *Am. J. Med.,* **62,** 707 (1977).

183. D. E. Wilson and R. S. Lees, *J. Clin. Invest.,* **51,** 1051 (1972).

184. P. Puska, J. M. Iacono, et al., *Lancet,* **1,** 1 (1983).

185. I. L. Rouse, L. J. Beilin, et al., *Lancet,* **1,** 5 (1983).

186. J. M. Iacono, M. W. Marshal, et al. *Prev. Med.,* **4,** 426 (1975).

187. A. I. Fleischman, M. L. Bierenbaum, et al., *J. Med. Soc. N.J.,* **76,** 181 (1979).

188. B. Stern, S. Heyden, et al., *Nutr. Metab.,* **24,** 137 (1980).

189. R. H. Rao, U. B. Rao, and S. G. Srikantia, *Clin. Exp. Hypertens.,* **3,** 27 (1981).

190. I. L. Rouse, B. K. Armstrong, and L. J. Beilin, *J. Hyper.,* **1,** 65 (1983).

191. F. G. McMahon, in *Management of Essential Hypertension; New Low Dose Era,* 2nd. Ed., Futura, Mt Kisco, NY, 1984, Chap. 2.

192. W. L. T. Addison, *Can. Med. Assoc. J.,* **18,** 282 (1928).

193. W. W. Priddle, *Can. Med. Assoc. J.,* **86,** 1 (1982).

194. G. R. Meneely and H. D. Battarbee, *Am. J. Cardiol.,* **38,** 768 (1976).

195. N. Sasaki, T. Mitsuhashi, and S. Fukushi, *Igaku Seibutsugaku,* **51,** 103 (1959).

196. J. Staesson, C. Bulpitt, R. Fagard, et al., "Four Urinary Cations and Blood Pressure-a Population Study of Two Belgian Towns," *International Symposium on Potassium, Blood Pressure and Cardiovascular Disease,* Excerpta Medica (in press) 1983.

197. K. T. Khaw and G. Rose, *Int. J. Epidemiol.,* **11,** 372 (1982).

198. H. G. Langford and R. L. Watson, "Electrolytes and Hypertension," in O. Paul, Ed., *Epidemiology and Control of Hypertension,* Stratton, New York, 1975.

199. R. L. Watson, H. G. Langford, J. D. Abernethy, et al., *Hypertension,* **2,** 93 (1980).

200. W. G. Walker, P. K. Whetlon, H. Saito, et al., *Hypertension,* **1,** 287 (1979).

201. C. J. Bulpitt, M. J. Shipley and A. Semnence, *Clin. Sci.,* **61,** 85s (1981).

202. F. Skrabal, J. Auboch, and H. Hortnagl, *Lancet,* **2,** 895 (1981).

203. T. B. Van Itallie and H. R. Kissileff, "Estimation of Satiating Efficiency of Dietary Fiber: Some Old Problems and a New Strategy, in *New Trends in Pathophysiology and Therapy of the Large Bowl,* L. Barbara M. Miglioli, and S. F. Phillips, Eds., Elsevier, Amsterdam, pp. 235–245.

204. P. Wilmshurst and J. C. W. Crawley, *Brit. J. Nutr.,* **44,** 1 (1980).

205. G. V. Vahouny, T. Roy, L. L. Gallo, J. A. Story, D. Kritchevsky, M. Cassidy, B. M. Grund, and C. R. Treadwell, *Am. J. Clin. Nutr.,* **31,** S208 (1978).

9

Clinical Aspects of Exercise and Diabetes Mellitus

STEPHEN H. SCHNEIDER, M.D.
and HASSAN KANJ, M.D.

UMDNJ-Rutgers Medical School, New Brunswick, New Jersey

Regular exercise is now widely recommended to patients with diabetes mellitus. Nevertheless, there are surprisingly few well-controlled studies demonstrating its beneficial effects and the specifics of an ideal exercise prescription have not been well established. We will discuss the potential benefits of exercise on glycemic control and its potential role in reducing the incidence of atherosclerosis in the diabetic population. We will also discuss some complications of exercise in diabetes and address the issue of developing specific exercise recommendations.

HISTORY

The therapeutic benefits of regular exercise have been recognized since prehistoric times. Hippocrates recognized its value for strengthening weakened muscles, hastening convalescence, and improving mental attitudes. Frequent and rapid walks were recommended to treat obesity. In addition, caution was advised in the resumption of strenuous exercise after prolonged rest (1).

The therapeutic usefulness of physical activity for patients with diabetes mellitus was suggested as early as 600 B.C. by the Indian physician Sushruta (2), and Celsus (30 B.C. to A.D. 50) prescribed exercise to patients with glycosuria (3), but it was not until the eighteenth century that the value of exercise became widely accepted in the west (4). In the preinsulin era, the therapeutic importance of physical exercise was emphasized by Bouchardat (5) and Trousseau (6) and subsequently supported by others (7–8).

It should be remembered that this early clinical impression of the beneficial effect of exercise was limited for the most part to patients with relatively mild type II diabetes, as patients with severe disease rarely survived. In this respect it is interesting to note that John Rollo in 1798 (10), on the basis of his experience with a population having more severe metabolic derangements, condemned exercise and prescribed total bed rest.

In the twentieth century, exercise has attracted growing attention as a means for improving metabolic control in patients with diabetes mellitus and was strongly advocated as a "cornerstone" of treatment by Joslin (11) and Katsch (12) at the beginning of the insulin era. Thus exercise became one of the three basic components of diabetes management along with diet and insulin. Nevertheless, it is only in recent years that controlled studies have been performed to clarify the role of exercise as a therapy for this disease.

CARBOHYDRATE METABOLISM DURING EXERCISE

To understand the interaction of exercise with the diabetic state, it is relevant to review the metabolic changes that occur during physical activity in normal man. In the resting state, skeletal muscle depends almost exclusively on the oxidation of free fatty acids as its main energy-yielding substrate. At the onset of mild to moderate exercise, muscle glycogen is the major fuel consumed, but shortly thereafter blood glucose uptake by muscle begins to increase progressively independent of changes in plasma insulin levels, rising from 7 to 20 times basal, depending on the intensity of the work performed. By 40 minutes of exercise, blood-borne glucose is responsible for 75 to 90% of the total carbohydrate consumed, reflecting a progressive decrease in the availability of muscle glycogen. During more prolonged exercise, the rate of glucose utilization peaks at 90 to 180 minutes and then declines slightly. At this time blood glucose accounts for 35 to 40% of the total fuel utilization, the rest being accounted for by oxidation of free fatty acids. Thus the overall pattern of fuel utilization during prolonged periods of mild to moderate exercise may be characterized as a triphasic response in which muscle glycogen, a combination of stored glycogen and blood glucose, and free fatty acids successively predominate as the major energy-yielding substrate (13,14).

To meet the increased glucose requirements of exercise, hepatic glucose output increases as soon as exercise begins. Initially most of the glucose comes from stored glycogen. Subsequently the relative contribution of hepatic gluconeogenesis to hepatic glucose output increases from 25% in the basal state to 45% during prolonged moderate exercise, a threefold rise in the absolute gluconeogenic rate. This equilibrium between glucose production and utilization will maintain plasma glucose within a remarkably narrow range for many hours. Eventually, however, glucose production fails to keep up with glucose utilization and plasma glucose levels slowly decline (15).

Upon cessation of exercise, glucose flux is directed towards rapid replenishment of glycogen stores (16) mediated in part by an increase in the insulin sensitivity of skeletal muscle (17). It is important to emphasize that these effects may persist for many hours following an exercise bout. The factors that modulate increased glucose uptake and insulin sensitivity after exercise are discussed elsewhere in this volume by Dr. Ruderman.

HORMONAL RESPONSES DURING EXERCISE

Control of the complex metabolic changes occurring during exercise is mediated by the well-integrated effects of the entire neuroendocrine system. With the onset of exercise, a decrease in circulating insulin level is observed (18), probably due primarily to an α-adrenergic inhibition of insulin secretion (19) which is more pronounced with prolonged or severe exercise (15). The decrease in plasma insulin levels may contribute to the increase in hepatic glucose production during exercise; however, it does not appear to be indispensable. Although the increase in peripheral uptake of glucose is not mediated by an increase in plasma insulin levels, animal experiments have demonstrated that in the complete absence of insulin, glucose uptake fails to increase during muscle contraction (20), suggesting that insulin may play a permissive role. This permissive effect of insulin is demonstrable in animal experiments at concentrations well below the concentration found in exercising healthy man (15,21) and lower than that found in most 24 hour insulin-withdrawn diabetic patients (22,23). Recently, Garetto and coworkers (24) showed that glucose utilization after high intensity exercise is enhanced despite the almost total absence of insulin in muscles which are severely glycogen depleted. Thus the role of permissive levels of plasma insulin in the enhanced glucose uptake of contracting skeletal muscle is not yet fully understood.

The importance of the counterregulatory hormones in maintaining plasma glucose levels during exercise also requires further study. It appears that the early decrease in the plasma insulin level sensitizes the liver to glucagon and epinephrine, allowing basal levels to contribute to an increase in hepatic glucose output (25–33). Later, as plasma glucose levels begin to decline, absolute elevations of epinephrine and glucagon occur which may further contribute to hepatic glucose output and may help to restrain peripheral glucose utilization. This counterregulatory hormonal response could be particularly important for the prevention of exercise-induced hypoglycemia during prolonged exercise or in the face of inappropriately high insulin levels.

ALTERATION OF CARBOHYDRATE METABOLISM DURING EXERCISE IN THE PRESENCE OF DEFICIENT INSULIN ACTIVITY

Severe insulin deficiency results in depletion of hepatic and skeletal muscle glycogen stores (34). However, the uptake of glucose by exercising muscle of insulin-withdrawn animals (35) and humans (23,36) is comparable to normal and the additional energy requirement is made up for by an increased utilization of free fatty acids (23,34). In addition, gluconeogenesis more rapidly becomes an important source of hepatic glucose output (37,38). Thus the overall effect of short-term exercise in patients with diabetes mellitus in poor metabolic control is comparable to that of prolonged exercise in normal man resulting in an accelerated metabolic adaptation.

EFFECTS OF EXERCISE ON GLUCOSE TOLERANCE AND GLYCEMIC CONTROL

It has been demonstrated that physical inactivity, even a few days of bed rest, can result in glucose intolerance and insulin resistance in normal man (39–41). However, epidemiologic studies comparing estimated habitual physical activity and glucose tolerance have yielded variable results. Mouratoff and coworkers (42) were able to show such an association in normal Eskimos; however, Montoye and coworkers (43) did not observe this relationship in a study of 10,000 normal persons in Tecumsch, Georgia, nor did Saltin and Lindgarde (44) in their study on middle-aged Scandinavian men.

Studies in animal models have consistently demonstrated enhanced glucose disposal and insulin sensitivity following physical training (45,46), and human studies have demonstrated similar findings in endurance athletes (47,48), obese subjects (49), and subjects with impaired glucose tolerance (50). While some of the improvement in insulin sensitivity may be related to weight loss, similar changes have been demonstrated in the absence of measurable changes in weight or adiposity (51–53). Koivisto and coworkers (54) suggested that the enhanced sensitivity may be due to increased binding of insulin to its receptors.

Effects of Exercise on Glycemic Control in Type I Diabetes Mellitus

Decreased insulin requirements during periods of increased physical activity have been frequently observed in patients with type I diabetes. Vranic and Berger (55) reported decreased insulin requirements in children with diabetes during summer camp and Marble and coworkers (56), Costill and coworkers (57), and Engerbretson (58) showed similar results following intensive physical training. The studies of Wallberg-Henriksson and coworkers (59) and De Fronzo and coworkers (60) confirmed these observations and demonstrated an associated improvement in insulin sensitivity as assessed by the glucose and insulin clamp techniques, respectively.

Surprisingly, improved glycemic control in patients with type I diabetes as a result of physical training has not yet been convincingly demonstrated. Thus Peterson and coworkers (61) found improved glycemic control in 10 patients with type I diabetes after 8 to 10 weeks of physical training, but did not control for simultaneous changes in dietary habits and insulin administration. Better controlled studies, such as those of Wallberg-Henriksson and coworkers (59) and DeFronzo and coworkers (60) have failed to demonstrate improved overall glycemic control despite significant improvements in insulin sensitivity. There are probably a variety of explanations for this apparent discrepancy. Improved insulin sensitivity might not necessarily result in improved glycemic control in insulin-deficient patients for whom the major clinical consideration is the timing and distribution of insulin action. Also, in many cases, the decrease in insulin dosage and increase in carbohydrate intake necessary to avoid exercise-induced hypoglycemia negate the beneficial effect of exercise on insulin sensitivity in the clinical setting.

Effects of Exercise on Glycemic Control in Patients with Type II Diabetes Mellitus

Studies of the beneficial effects of exercise training in patients with type II diabetes present a more optimistic picture. Insulin resistance is an important pathogenetic factor in the glucose intolerance of a large number of patients with early and mild type II diabetes, and timing and distribution of exogenous insulin administration are less important.

That exercise can lower the plasma glucose concentration in

such patients was initially demonstrated by Allen and coworkers (7) before the insulin era. Saltin and coworkers (50) demonstrated a modest improvement in fasting hyperglycemia and glucose tolerance after 5 months of physical training assessed 3 days after the last exercise bout. Ruderman and coworkers (62) showed a small improvement in intravenous but not oral glucose tolerance after 6 weeks of physical training in six patients with type II diabetes evaluated 2 weeks after the last exercise bout. Bogardus and coworkers (63) demonstrated improvement in glycemic control and glucose disposal in obese patients with type II diabetes but concomitant weight reduction makes the independent effects of exercise difficult to isolate.

Acute Effects of Exercise vs. Physical Training

Although most studies demonstrate a modest improvement in glycemic control during programs of regular exercise training, it is not clear to what extent these changes are due to the residual effects of the individual exercise bouts or to the improved state of aerobic fitness per se. Improved glucose disposal following a single bout of intensive exercise has been repeatedly demonstrated in association with enhanced insulin sensitivity, and this can affect meal-related glycemic excursion. For example, Caron and coworkers (64) in a study of patients with type I diabetes showed that exercise after breakfast resulted in markedly decreased glycemic excursions after lunch. This effect of exercise is transient, lasting hours to a few days, depending on the intensity and duration of physical activity (62, 65–68). We have assessed the effects of 6 weeks of physical training on a group of 20 sedentary men with type II diabetes on a weight maintenance diet (68). Improved glycemic control was confirmed by a decrease in levels of glycosylated hemoglobin. Oral glucose tolerance performed 3 days after the last exercise bout showed only minimal improvement, but 12 hours after the last exercise bout glucose tolerance was significantly enhanced (Figure 9-1). There was no measurable decrease in the improved state of aerobic fitness as assessed by VO_{2max} over these 72 hours of inactivity.

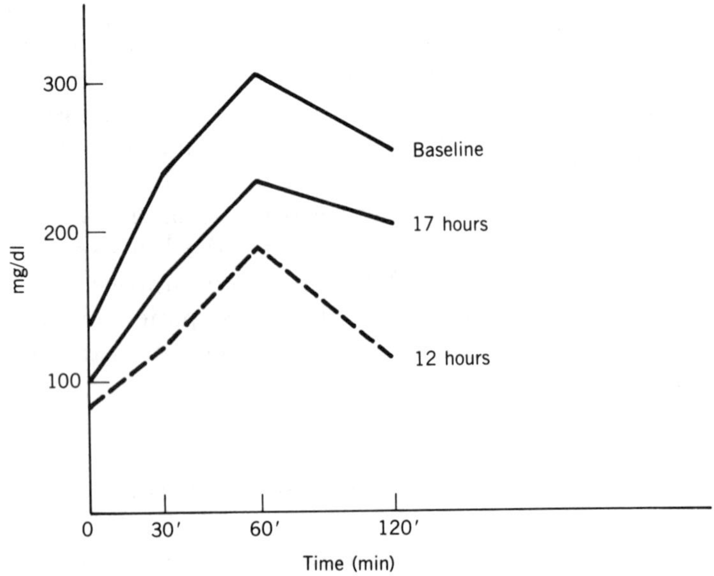

Figure 9-1. Glucose tolerance following a single exercise bout in a diabetic patient.

These data are consistent with the concept that improved glycemic control was the result of the summed effects of the individual exercise bouts and not of the state of enhanced aerobic fitness per se. Recent studies by Skor and coworkers (67) suggest that improved aerobic fitness may potentiate and prolong the metabolic effects of an acute exercise bout. Thus physical training may play an indirect role in enhancing glucose tolerance. These observations may help to reconcile the results of studies in which glucose tolerance was determined at various times relative to the last exercise bout and also emphasize the importance of the frequency of exercise sessions for the overall glycemic response.

The mechanisms of improved glucose tolerance following an acute exercise bout require more investigation. They may include production of local humoral factors (69), changes in insulin receptor number or affinity (54), or non-receptor-mediated alterations in tissue responsiveness to insulin (70). Better understanding of what determines this response will be a major step towards optimizing recommendations for an exercise prescription.

POTENTIAL BENEFITS OF REGULAR EXERCISE ON THE RISK OF ATHEROSCLEROTIC CARDIOVASCULAR DISEASE IN DIABETES MELLITUS

Diabetes mellitus is a major risk factor for atherosclerosis (71,72). Epidemiologic studies have established that cerebrovascular, coronary, and peripheral artery disease are more common in diabetes and occur at an earlier age (72,73). In addition, diabetes mellitus eliminates the relative protection from atherosclerosis possessed by premenopausal women (72–76). Coronary heart disease mortality is approximately doubled for subjects with impaired glucose tolerance (72). This increased risk appears to be independent of the absolute level of glycemic control or whether the patient is treated by diet, oral agents, or insulin. Despite the increased incidence and wide distribution of atherosclerotic lesions in diabetes, the histology of the lesion appears to be almost identical to that found in men without diabetes (77). While often considered the major complication of type II diabetes, atherosclerotic disease is also a major problem in type I diabetes. For example, Crall and Roberts (78) have demonstrated significant coronary artery disease in patients with type I diabetes autopsied at age 19 to 38 whose onset of disease was in childhood. This problem may become increasingly important as our improved ability to treat the complications of microvascular disease allows patients with type I diabetes to achieve longer lifespans.

Protective Effects of Regular Physical Activity on Atherosclerosis

Table 9-1 lists risk factors for atherosclerotic cardiovascular disease (ASCVD) in type II diabetes. Animal studies suggest a protective effect of exercise training on ASCVD. Myocardial in-

Table 9-1. Risk Factors for ASCVD in Type II Diabetes

Glucose intolerance
Hyperinsulinemia
Dyslipidemia
Hypertension
Hypercoagulable state
Decreased fitness
Obesity
Psychological stress

farction size has been shown to be smaller in trained young animals following experimental coronary occlusion (79). Other studies demonstrated an increase in coronary artery diameter (80), coronary collateral circulation (81), and in muscle capillary to fiber ratio (82) following regular physical exercise. Kramsch and his colleagues (83) have shown that exercise markedly retards the development of atherosclerosis in monkeys maintained on a high cholesterol diet.

In humans, epidemiologic studies suggest that endurance-type exercise diminishes both the mortality and morbidity from atherosclerotic vascular disease in normal populations and patients with diabetes (84–90). In a study of Harvard graduates, Paffenberger and coworkers (86) noted that the incidence of first heart attacks was significantly lower in individuals with the greatest degree of physical activity. The protective effect of exercise was also seen among cigarette smokers, hypertensives, and patients with diabetes. Athletes were at a low risk for coronary heart disease only if they had continued vigorous activity into adulthood. In the Framingham study (90), coronary heart disease incidence and mortality after 14 years were inversely related to a physical activity index in men. This also was independent of age, blood pressure, smoking, and plasma cholesterol levels.

While the reason for the increased incidence of atherosclerosis in diabetes is not fully understood, a number of risk factors known to be associated with cardiovascular disease are often found in patients with diabetes and may be favorably influenced by regular exercise. In particular, the contributions and interactions of hyperglycemia, insulin resistance, hyperlipidemia, the hypercoagulable state, and obesity to the atherosclerotic process are under investigation (91,92).

Glucose Intolerance

The role of glucose intolerance and hyperglycemia per se as a risk factor for atherosclerosis is unclear. A review of 11 prospective studies by Stamler and Stamler (93) failed to confirm an increased risk of atherosclerosis in the presence of glucose intolerance. On the other hand, Fuller and his associates (94) found that coronary heart disease mortality was approximately doubled for subjects with impaired glucose tolerance independent of other risk factors, and the Framingham study data (72) suggest that even mild hyperglycemia is associated with a doubling of risk for coronary artery disease. Surprisingly, little additional risk is associated with development of overt diabetes mellitus.

Because of the large population of patients with glucose intolerance it is important that more work be done to investigate possible mechanisms by which mild hyperglycemia might contribute to atherosclerotic risk. One such mechanism would be nonenzymatic glycosylation of proteins. This may contribute directly by altering the connective tissue and cellular components in the vessel wall and indirectly by exacerbating a number of other risk factors. For example, nonenzymatic glycosylation of HDL and LDL apoproteins (95) and fibrinogen (96,97) has recently been demonstrated.

Hyperinsulinemia

Many patients with type II diabetes have significant hyperinsulinemia as part of their disease or as a result of treatment with exogenous insulin. In addition, many patients with type I diabetes are being treated aggressively with insulin, in an attempt to maintain near normal blood glucose levels, and have elevated plasma free insulin levels for large parts of the day.

Hyperinsulinemia and insulin resistance have been proposed as potential risk factors for atherosclerosis (98,99). Animal studies have clearly demonstrated that exogenous insulin administration worsens atherosclerotic lesions of the aorta (100) and may even prevent the regression of experimental atherosclerosis in chickens (101).

Epidemiologic studies have revealed that subjects with disease of coronary (102–109), cerebral (110), or peripheral (109, 111,112) arteries have elevated insulin responses to an oral glucose load when compared to subjects without evidence of vascular disease. Furthermore, Santen and colleagues (113) found a higher insulin to glucose ratio in patients with atherosclerosis, suggesting decreased insulin sensitivity. In addition three prospective studies, the Helsinki policemen study (114), the Paris study (115), and the Busselton-Australia study (116), have shown a strong correlation between insulin levels and ischemic heart disease. Insulin could act by altering metabolic pathways in vascular cells or by stimulating the growth of vascular smooth muscle cells (117,118).

Regular exercise has been shown to result in decreased insulin levels in normal subjects, obese subjects, and subjects with impaired glucose tolerance (119–122). Furthermore, it has been shown to diminish insulin requirements in insulin-treated patients primarily by enhancing insulin sensitivity (55–58).

The effect of exercise on insulin levels in patients with type II diabetes is still controversial. Minuk and coworkers (123) failed to show a decrease in the elevated resting insulin levels in obese patients with diabetes after exercise despite a significant decrease in plasma glucose levels. Our own data and that of others suggest that improvements in glycemic control and glucose tolerance associated with exercise in patients with type II diabetes occur in the face of unchanged insulin levels consistent with improved insulin sensitivity. In patients taking insulin this would be expected to result in decreased insulin requirements. Nevertheless, substantial reductions of endogenous plasma insulin levels in patients with type II diabetes mellitus in association with exercise training may not occur in the absence of significant weight reduction, although there may be a small subgroup of hyperinsulinemic patients for whom regular exercise training results in a significant reduction in plasma insulin levels, especially after a meal.

Dyslipidemias

Hyperlipidemia is a common finding in patients with diabetes. The pattern depends on the severity of the metabolic derangement, the type of diabetes, and the treatment modality. While a variety of patterns have been noted, studies of patients with type II diabetes most commonly demonstrate elevation of triglyceride and cholesterol levels and lower than normal levels of HDL cholesterol (124–127). In contrast, studies of well-controlled insulin-treated patients with type I diabetes have most often demonstrated normal or elevated HDL cholesterol levels (128,129).

Cross-sectional (130) and longitudinal studies (131–136) in normal subjects have demonstrated that regular exercise can favorably alter plasma lipids, presumably decreasing cardiovascular risk. Plasma triglyceride and VLDL levels are particularly sensitive to the lipid-lowering effects of regular exercise, whereas a decrease in plasma cholesterol levels has not been consistently demonstrated (136–140). While the atherogenic potential of VLDL particles is unclear, VLDL particles of patients with diabetes may be altered to become more atherogenic. It was shown recently that glucosylation of LDL particles to an extent similar to that seen in diabetes slows their catabolism (141). A similar mechanism for VLDL particles may be a contributing factor to their atherogenicity. Thus lowering of VLDL by regular exercise may exert a beneficial effect.

Ruderman and colleagues (62) in their study on patients with type II diabetes undergoing physical training noted a significant decrease in plasma triglyceride levels and a much smaller decrease in plasma cholesterol level, and similar results were noted in our study of 20 sedentary patients with type II diabetes participating in a regular training program. Plasma cholesterol and HDL cholesterol levels did not change significantly. In a larger clinical study of 108 patients followed in our diabetes exercise program, an average fall in plasma triglyceride level of 15% from the basal level was found over 3 months with no change in cholesterol and HDL cholesterol levels.

The mechanisms of the lipid-lowering effect of physical training are complex and many studies are difficult to interpret because of the confounding effects of concomitant weight reduction. Decreased hepatic glycogen stores and hepatic glucose uptake during the postexercise recovery period may mediate a reduced VLDL production by the liver through lack of substrate (130). Moreover, an increase of lipoprotein lipase in skeletal muscles and adipose tissue has been demonstrated after a 2 km race in trained subjects (142).

The time course of changes in plasma triglyceride levels suggests that, as with glucose, much of the benefits of exercise training are due to the summed effects of the individual exercise bouts (143–145). Holoszy and coworkers (137) and Cullinane and coworkers (144) demonstrated a decrease in plasma triglyceride levels after a bout of intensive exercise which returned to basal levels over 48 to 72 hours. In our studies a significant decrease in plasma triglyceride level was consistently noted 12 hours after a typical exercise training bout, but 72 hours later the improvement was no longer measurable (Figure 9-2).

Elevations of plasma HDL cholesterol level during physical training in normal man may be linked to alterations in VDL metabolism (130,146–148). However, attempts to elevate plasma HDL cholesterol level with exercise alone may require exercise of longer duration and greater intensity than is usually recommended (136,138). For this and possibly other reasons, exercise training has not been consistently found to result in elevated HDL cholesterol levels in patients with diabetes mellitus.

Hypertension

Hypertension is more common in the diabetic population. Epidemiologic studies (149–153) indicate that active individuals have significantly lower systolic and diastolic blood pressure at rest than their less active peers, and exercise training has been shown by many but not all investigators to lower blood pressure at rest in normotensive and hypertensive subjects (154–160).

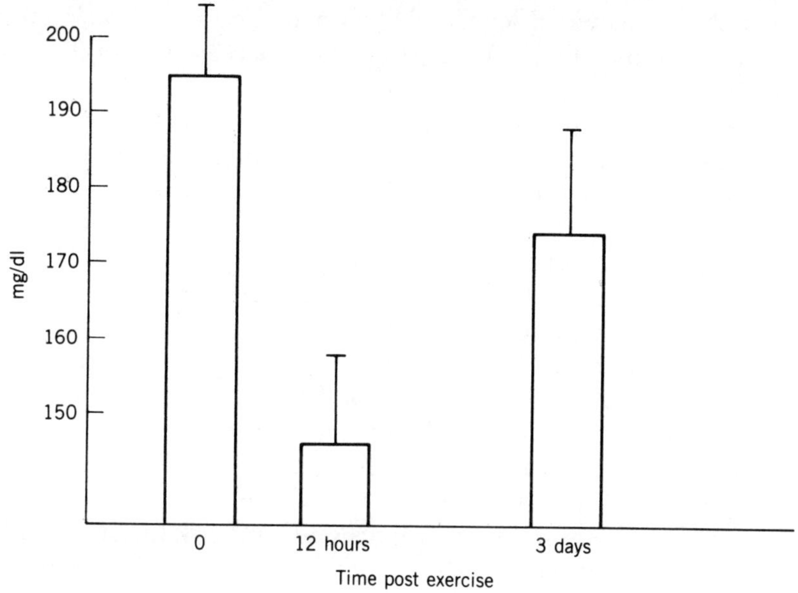

Figure 9-2. Effect of a single exercise bout on plasma triglyceride level.

In our own studies exercise and diet therapy have been quite effective in reducing the blood pressure of hypertensive patients with type II diabetes, with a mean reduction of 10–15 mmHg of diastolic blood pressure following 4 months of exercise therapy. The mechanisms by which exercise reduces blood pressure are poorly understood at the present time; the lower level of sympathetic activity demonstrated after training (161,162) may play a role. It is interesting to note, however, that patients with type II diabetes who are hypertensive are more likely to be hyperinsulinemic and the patients with the best blood pressure response to exercise training are those in whom the plasma insulin level decreases (163).

Hypercoagulable State

An area of increasing interest is the role of the coagulation system in the vascular complications of diabetes mellitus. Patients with diabetes suffer from a ''hypercoagulable'' state. This is associated with elevated levels of fibrinogen and factor VIII complex activity, platelet hyperaggregability, increased thromboxane and decreased prostacycline synthesis, and a depressed fibrinolytic response to a variety of stimuli (164–166). It is not yet clear to what degree these changes are related to metabolic control and to what extent they are the result of vascular injury.

The association between the hypercoagulable state and atherosclerosis is also unresolved. Aggregation of platelets at the endothelial wall releases growth factors that may enhance smooth muscle proliferation and this provides one theoretical mechanism for acceleration of the atherosclerotic process (167). It is relevant to note that pigs deficient in factor VIII activity appear to be resistant to the induction of atherosclerotic lesions (168), although this has been recently challenged (169). Wilhelmsen and colleagues (170) in a study of 792 men found that elevated levels of fibrinogen are associated with a significant risk for both stroke and myocardial infarction. The APTT V_{max}, the maximum rate of fibrin polymer formation during the activated partial thromboplastin time, is believed to be a sensitive measure of the hypercoagulable state, and a recent retrospective study has shown elevations of the APTT V_{max} in patients with premature coronary heart disease (171).

In normal man exercise results in improved fibrinolysis and decreased levels of factor VIII VWF activity and may favorably affect other components of the coagulation system (172–177). Our patients with type II diabetes had elevated APTT V_{max} and PT V_{max} and impaired fibrinolysis. Both these abnormalities improved after 6 weeks of exercise training (unpublished data).

Aerobic Exercise Performance

Most studies of patients with type I diabetes have demonstrated normal levels of aerobic fitness, as measured by the VO_{2max}, compared to appropriate controls in the absence of significant autonomic neuropathy (57,178,179). In patients with type II diabetes, however, Saltin and coworkers (50), Ruderman and coworkers (62), and Rubler (180) demonstrated an unexpectedly low VO_{2max}. However, none of these reports include a detailed assessment of the cardiovascular and neurological status of the patients, or their recreational and occupational activities. Our studies have confirmed this observation in patients with similar recreational and work activities to control subjects. A decrease in VO_{2max} could result from changes in the central circulation, autonomic nervous system dysfunction, or changes in skeletal muscle (181). Although we did not find clinical evidence of cardiovascular disease and autonomic neuropathy in our patients and only a few had clearly abnormal R-R interval variation, more subtle abnormalities of these systems cannot be excluded. Recent studies by Saltin and colleagues (44,50) have revealed a decreased activity of oxidative enzymes as well as abnormalities of fiber type area distribution, capillary density, and staining characteristics in skeletal muscle of patients with "chemical diabetes" and impaired glucose tolerance.

Whether the decreased VO_{2max} in patients with type II diabetes is secondary to the metabolic abnormalities or is independent of and precedes them remains to be established. Saltin and colleagues (44) demonstrated a similar decrease in VO_{2max} in subjects with impaired glucose tolerance without overt diabetes mellitus when compared to appropriate controls with normal glucose tolerance. This suggests that the abnormality in aerobic exercise performance could precede the major metabolic disturbance of the diabetic state. Interestingly, when these subjects were followed over a 3 year period, none of 52 subjects who engaged in a program of long-term aerobic training developed overt diabetes, whereas 15% of the untrained subjects did. These observations raise the possibility that programs designed to increase aerobic work capacity may protect a subgroup of the population with glucose intolerance from progressing to overt diabetes mellitus.

Weight Control

Exercise can be an effective addition to weight control regimens (63). Not only are extra calories consumed during exercise but under certain circumstances metabolic rates may remain increased for several hours after cessation of physical activity. On the other hand, in our experience, minimal weight reduction is achieved by exercise programs of modest intensity unless caloric intake is simultaneously controlled.

Psychological Stress

Chronic illnesses such as diabetes mellitus may be associated with significant pyschological stress. Stress in turn may worsen glucose intolerance and be an additional risk factor for accelerated atherosclerosis (182). Repeated studies have revealed improvements in some psychological parameters with regular exercise, especially reduction in perception and response to psychological stress (161,183). Depression and anxiety are particularly likely to improve. Unfortunately, in our experience, potentially detrimental type A personality traits are not altered by exercise training.

OSTEOPOROSIS AND BONE MASS IN DIABETES MELLITUS

Insulin stimulates the uptake of amino acids in bone (184), exerts a stimulatory effect on collagen synthesis in bone organ cultures (185), and stimulates intestinal calcium absorption (186). Thus diabetes and insulin deficiency may contribute to osteoporosis in laboratory animals (187) and man (188).

Animal studies have demonstrated that rats with diabetes develop a negative calcium balance (189–192) which may be due to an insulin correctable reduction in serum 1,25 di(OH)vitamin D concentrations (192). Furthermore, experimental diabetes in rats induced by alloxan causes loss of bone mass (187).

In 1949 Albright and Reifenstein (193) reported the occurrence of osteoporosis in patients with longstanding and poorly controlled diabetes. Menczel and coworkers (194) reported a 22% incidence of proximal hip fractures in patients with diabetes, thus emphasizing its importance. Reduced bone mass is confirmed in patients with type I and type II diabetes in some studies (195–199) but not in others (200–205). Levin and colleagues (195) studied a large series of patients with diabetes and found a significant loss of bone mass as compared to controls. The decrease in bone mass did not correlate with the duration of diabetes and the greatest decrease was noted in patients receiving oral agents. He proposed that the diabetic osteopenia is completely or partially reversible by insulin treatment. One factor contributing to the variable findings in many studies is the effect of body weight, as obesity appears to exert a protective effect on skeletal mass (205). Thus obese patients with type II diabetes may be less likely to develop significant bone loss.

Exercise, particularly when weight bearing is involved, has been shown to protect skeletal mass in postmenopausal women and delay the onset of senile osteoporosis. This has been demonstrated in control subjects, for example, athletes, and in postmenopausal females with and without osteoporosis (206,207). However, no direct evidence of the effects of exercise training on bone mass in patients with diabetes is available.

COMPLICATIONS OF EXERCISE THERAPY

Metabolic

Hypoglycemia. Hypoglycemia is a frequent and sometimes serious complication of exercise in insulin-treated patients. It is not seen in patients treated with diet alone and is rarely encountered with sulfonylureas. The magnitude of the hypoglycemic response is dependent on the initial plasma glucose level, duration and intensity of exercise, and plasma insulin concentration. It should be noted that patients with diabetes sometimes experience symptoms of hypoglycemia when their plasma glucose concentrations fall rapidly to the normal or even mildly hyperglycemic range during an exercise bout (208). Hypoglycemia may also be observed several hours after exercise (56). This delayed effect is consistent with the increased insulin sensitivity which persists for hours following an exercise bout.

Type I patients treated with continuous subcutaneous insulin infusion (CSII) with a portable pump may be at an even greater risk for hypoglycemia. Although Trovati and coworkers (209) did not find an increased risk of hypoglycemia in patients treated with CSII during exercise, Koivisto and colleagues (210) found that CSII-treated patients were at increased risk. One obvious difference between these studies was that exercise was performed shortly after a premeal insulin bolus in the latter. Poussier and coworkers (211) demonstrated that exercise-induced hypoglycemia in CSII-treated patients was related to the usual postmeal increment in the rate of insulin administration. Maintaining the insulin infusion at the basal rate when exercise followed a meal usually prevented the hypoglycemic response.

The reasons for hypoglycemia during and shortly after exercise are not fully understood. In addition to the increase in insulin sensitivity two possible mechanisms have been emphasized:

1. An accelerated absorption of depot insulin during exercise of underlying muscles (212–214).
2. An inability to lower plasma insulin concentrations to levels obtained in normal subjects during exercise because exogenous insulin administration results in an imbalance between hepatic glucose production and peripheral glucose utilization (55,215–218).

Although these mechanisms may sometimes contribute to hypoglycemia during exercise, altering the injection site only occasionally results in amelioration of the tendency for hypoglycemia (219–220). In addition, Chisholm and coworkers (221) have demonstrated that moderate hyperinsulinemia is insufficient to restrain hepatic glucose output during exercise in normal subjects and it has been repeatedly demonstrated that maintaining the basal level of insulin by its intravenous administration during exercise does not predictably result in hypoglycemia in patients with type I diabetes (215,216,222,223). Thus the pathogenesis of hypoglycemia during exercise in many patients remains poorly understood.

Recent studies of patients with type I diabetes who have suffered severe and recurrent hypoglycemia during intensive insulin therapy indicate that some of these individuals suffer from an impaired glucagon and epinephrine response to insulin-induced hypoglycemia (208,224–231). These hormones may play a role in maintaining hepatic glucose output and restraining peripheral glucose utilization in the face of relative hyperinsulinemia, and in some instances their deficiency could contribute to the hypoglycemic tendency.

The role of various commonly used pharmacologic agents in exercise-induced hypoglycemia requires more studies. Beta-adrenergic blocking agents used in the treatment of hypertension and coronary artery disease might aggravate exercise-induced hypoglycemia, especially in the subgroup of patients with an impaired glucagon response (232). Recently, Ferriere and colleagues (233) demonstrated an increased glucose disposal rate in patients with diabetes treated with captopril, and others have shown that prostaglandin synthetase inhibitors, such as indomethacin, can impair hepatic glycogenolysis (234).

Clearly exercise-induced hypoglycemia in insulin-treated patients with diabetes remains a major concern and is a fertile area for future research. Some general recommendations of practical value in avoiding this problem are listed in Table 9-2.

Hyperglycemia and Ketosis. Exercise under conditions of poor metabolic control may actually worsen hyperglycemia and

Table 9-2. Prevention of Exercise-Related Hypoglycemia

1. Decrease dose of insulin
2. Increase CHO consumption (15-30 g/30 min)
3. Inject away from most active muscle groups
4. Do not exercise shortly after an insulin injection. Exercising in the morning before your a.m injection may yield the best benefits in plasma glucose with the lowest risk of hypoglycemia.

occasionally precipitate ketosis in patients with type I diabetes (22,235–240). A similar but usually less severe problem can occur in patients with type II diabetes. In these patients, low effective plasma insulin levels together with elevated levels of the counterregulatory hormones, glucagon and epinephrine, result in excessive hepatic glucose production and ketogenesis. In addition, perhaps because of the severe insulin deficiency in such patients, the utilization of glucose and ketone bodies by exercising muscle is diminished. Fasting plasma glucose levels can be used for clinical purposes to assess the probability of this response. In general, a fasting plasma glucose level greater than 250 mg/dl is associated with metabolic deterioration during moderately intense exercise, whereas most patients with fasting plasma glucose less than 200 mg/dl demonstrate a hypoglycemic effect. In addition, in our studies we found a greater decrease in glycosylated hemoglobin levels after 6 weeks of training in patients with fasting plasma glucose levels below 200 mg/dl at entry into the program when compared to patients with glucose levels greater than 200 mg/dl (Figure 9-3). This may have an impact on the selection of patients for such training programs.

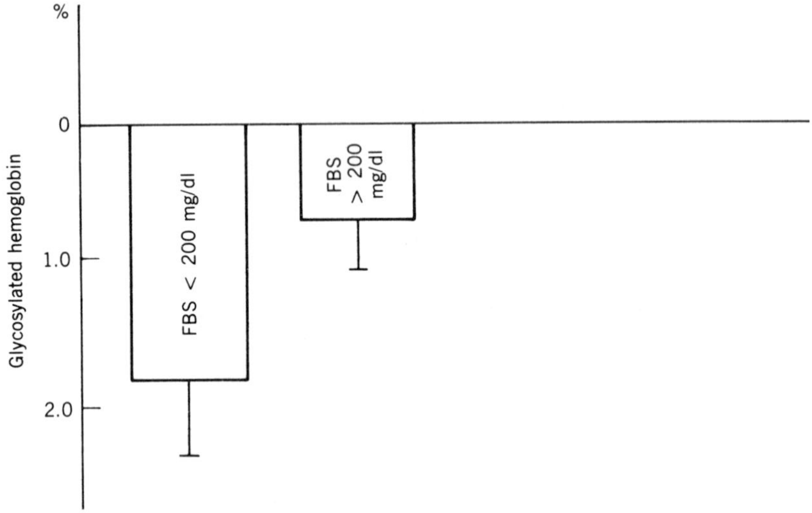

Figure 9-3. Imrovement of HbA_1 with regular exercise—relationship to fasting blood sugar levels.

Hyperkalemia. Transient hyperkalemia occurs during intensive exercise and resolves with recovery both in normals and in patients with diabetes mellitus. Both α- and β-adrenergic receptors appear to play important, but opposite, roles in modulating the "physiologic" hyperkalemia of exercise. α-adrenergic blocking agents decrease the rise in plasma potassium level and β-adrenergic blocking agents cause a sustained elevation of plasma potassium level during recovery (241).

Additional factors of particular relevance to patients with diabetes may substantially increase the risk of significant hyperkalemia. These include insulin deficiency, exaggerated levels of counterregulatory hormones, hyperglycemia, autonomic neuropathy, hyporeninemic hypoaldosteronism, and metabolic acidosis.

Although this has not been noted as a serious clinical problem in the past, the risk of hyperkalemia during exercise needs to be reevaluated as more patients with longstanding diabetes become involved in athletics and exercise programs and as the use of drugs which may exacerbate hyperkalemia, such as β-adrenergic blocking agents and captopril, increases.

Potential Vascular Complications of Exercise in Diabetes

Microvascular. There is some concern that moderate to heavy physical activity could contribute to the worsening of microvascular lesions in diabetes. Empirical observations of acceleration of retinopathy during exercise training are well known, but no controlled studies are available. The risk of exercise for those patients with established proliferative retinopathy is a major problem. Exercise at very high levels of intensity, isometric exercises, and exercise that requires Valsalva-type maneuvers, have been associated with subsequent retinal hemorrhage. Possible mechanisms include the hemodynamic changes induced by exercise as well as the increased levels of epinephrine and growth hormone. It is clear that exercise results in a transient increase in proteinuria in some normal and most diabetic patients. This is generally proportional to the intensity of exercise and the systolic blood pressure achieved and is probably due to altered renal hemodynamics (242). Whether these hemodynamic changes could lead to long-term detrimental results on the microvasculature is unknown, but the clear relationship between sustained systolic hypertension and renal and retinal microvascular disease makes it prudent to be cautious in this regard.

Macrovascular. The incidence of occult coronary artery disease is considerable in patients with type II diabetes. Waller and Roberts (243) in their study on 275 necropsy patients with diabetes mellitus found a higher incidence of significant narrowing of the left main coronary arteries when compared to controls matched with respect to age, sex, incidence of hypertension, and mean plasma cholesterol levels. Severe left main coronary artery narrowing occurred most frequently in patients whose onset of diabetes was between ages 16 and 30 years. In our own clinic 8% of the patients referred for exercise with no history or physical findings to suggest coronary artery disease are found to have clinically significant ischemia during exercise testing. The haphazard recommendation of unsupervised exercise to this high risk population is therefore not advisable. In our opinion all patients over the age of 40 or those with diabetes of more than 10 years duration at any age require careful evaluation prior to recommending exercise. The majority of older patients or patients with longstanding disease will require a specific exercise prescription and some monitoring of their cardiovascular response.

Miscellaneous Problems

A number of other potential problems must be considered in patients with diabetes mellitus undergoing exercise programs. A major concern is the diabetic foot. Patients with significant sensory loss in the feet should probably avoid exercises such as jogging, and those patients who choose to engage in an intensive running program should be seen by a podiatrist and provided with proper footwear.

Silberberg (244) found a positive correlation between degenerative joint disease and diabetes mellitus in autopsy studies. This was also demonstrated by Waine and coworkers (245). The mechanism is still unclear, but neuropathy and vasculopathy were postulated as a cause (246). Thus exercise that results in repeated joint trauma should be limited for patients with diabetes mellitus.

Some patients, especially those who are not well controlled and those with autonomic neuropathy, are prone to dehydration on warm days. Untrained patients may also have an increased incidence of postexercise hypotension after prolonged intense exercise. We generally recommend that patients with significant autonomic neuropathy abstain from intensive exercise or competitive sports (247).

THE EXERCISE PRESCRIPTION

Previously sedentary patients over the age of 40 or patients with longstanding diabetes should undergo some form of formal exercise testing prior to the recommendation of any but the most modest exercise program. This will help to detect occult coronary artery disease and is extremely useful in formulating specific exercise regimens. After a thorough evaluation an exercise prescription should be given including type of exercise, duration, frequency, intensity, and time of day.

Type of Exercise

Most programs of exercise therapy for patients with diabetes mellitus emphasize aerobic-type activities, such as swimming, cycling, and brisk walking. Although it is commonly believed that aerobic exercises are most effective in influencing metabolic abnormalities, recent studies suggest that power exercises, such as weight lifting, also result in significant improvements in glucose disposal (248). The increased glucose disposal appears to be related to the greater muscle mass in these subjects, as opposed to aerobic exercise where the improvement is based on greater efficiency of glucose disposal in muscle. It is not at all clear at present that these exercises should be discouraged, especially for younger patients with no serious vascular complications of their disease.

For older patients, however, and those with proliferative retinopathy, very high intensity exercise with its associated systolic hypertension and cardiovascular stress are ill-advised. Strenuous calisthetics and excessive isometric, stretching, and squatting maneuvers should also be discouraged.

Frequency

As discussed earlier many of the effects of a training program on glucose and lipid metabolism are related to the summed effects of the acute exercise bouts and are relatively transient. In general, the greater the frequency of exercise the greater the metabolic effect. In our studies we have found a frequency of three times a week to be the minimum required for consistent glycemic improvement. In eight patients whose glycosylated hemoglobin levels fell during thrice weekly exercise, deterioration of control was noted when we increased the intensity of exercise but decreased the frequency to twice weekly. This occurred despite the fact that these patients maintained their VO_{2max} at the same level.

Intensity and Duration

The effects of various intensities and durations of exercise on subsequent metabolic effects is not well worked out. It is not known if there are threshold levels of intensity and duration necessary for metabolic effects or if the total work performed is the major consideration. Older studies by Maehlum and Pruett (249) suggest that at work intensities of 50% VO_{2max} or greater, total work may be the most important determinant of the subsequent effect on glucose disposal but at less than 30% VO_{2max} no effect was noted. Other metabolic parameters may have different intensity and duration requirements. For example, increases in HDL cholesterol level have generally been noted with high intensity work loads for prolonged periods of time while changes in fibrinolysis appear to require work of sufficient intensity to generate metabolic acidosis. More information is clearly required to clarify these issues and it is likely that recommendations should vary depending on the specific goals of therapy.

In general, we have found a duration of at least 30 minutes per session to be satisfactory. Multiple brief rest periods of less than 90 seconds appear to have no impact on cardiovascular or metabolic effects as long as the total work time is kept constant. It appears reasonable in view of the lack of specific data to recommend an exercise intensity of 50–70% VO_{2max} for most patients based on the potential benefits and relative risks. In our experience this is most easily prescribed in terms of heart rate, which patients can be easily taught to monitor on their own. A rough target pulse can be obtained with the following formula:

$$\text{target pulse} = 0.5 \text{ to } 0.7\,(\text{maximal heart rate} - \text{rest heart rate}) + \text{rest heart rate}$$

Use of such formulas requires determination of true resting heart rate taken by the patient prior to getting out of bed in the morning. It should be noted that standard tables of maximal heart rate based on normal populations correlate poorly with maximal heart rate in patients with diabetes mellitus. We have often found a maximal heart rate 15 to 20% lower in patients with type II diabetes mellitus than their age-matched controls in the absence of clinically evident neuropathy or coronary heart disease. Autonomic neuropathy or sympatholytic drugs may further impair maximal heart rate and aerobic exercise performance. The exercise program is usually initiated at the lower target pulse and gradually increased to the desired target pulse over 2 to 3 weeks. Thereafter the intensity of exercise is slowly increased in order to maintain the same submaximal target pulse, resulting in a smooth progression of exercise intensity.

In addition to heart rate, the blood pressure response to exercise should be considered. Some normotensive patients develop severe systolic hypertension at surprisingly low work intensities.

It is probably prudent to limit exercise intensities to prevent systolic blood pressure from exceeding 180 mmHg for prolonged periods of time, especially in patients with established microvascular disease.

Time of Day

Little is known about the relative effects of a standard exercise done at different times of the day. In general, the major determinant of time of exercise is patient convenience. Because of the relatively transient effects of exercise on glucose disposal it is likely that exercise done in the early morning prior to breakfast would have the greatest impact on glycemic excursions throughout the day. Timing decisions are particularly difficult for patients with brittle type I diabetes. In these patients consistency of exercise timing and intensity from day to day may be the most important consideration. A reasonable recommendation would be to have a small snack on arising, exercise, and then take the daily insulin injection followed by breakfast. This regimen avoids problems of altered insulin absorption. Exercise late in the evening is often difficult to manage and can result in early morning hypoglycemia.

SELECTION OF PARTICIPANTS FOR AN EXERCISE PROGRAM

Supervised programs of exercise training for patients with diabetes mellitus are expensive and labor intensive. It is therefore necessary to attempt to identify subgroups of patients particularly likely to benefit from such programs as well as those for whom such programs are not indicated. Our own studies suggest that some metabolic and psychosocial profiles may be helpful in this respect. Patients who have demonstrated the best responses to exercise training in terms of glycemic control tend to have the following characteristics:

1. Type II diabetes mellitus
2. Poor initial aerobic fitness
3. Fasting plasma glucose levels less than 200 mg/dl
4. A well maintained or elevated plasma insulin level following a glucose challenge

Type I patients with difficulty in controlling their diabetes do especially poorly in exercise programs in our experience and often demonstrate metabolic deterioration. Recent studies have demonstrated that it may be possible to predict which patients are at greatest risk for unexpected hypoglycemia during programs of intensified insulin therapy (226). Similar attempts should be made to identify patients with type I diabetes most likely to have problems during an exercise training program.

Psychosocial factors in our studies have been highly predictive of patient's compliance in intensive outpatient programs involving exercise training (250). In general, self-referred patients and female patients have done particularly well. It is interesting that physicians in our community are more likely to refer male patients to an exercise program despite the poorer likelihood of good outcome.

Type A personality traits are a strong predictor of failure in a program if the patient is physician-referred. It should be noted that educational or economic level has had little impact on the eventual success in our own exercise training program.

Exercise training results in a complex interaction with the diabetic state. For many patients with type II diabetes it can be used as an effective adjunct to dietary therapy to obtain better glycemic control and improve the risk factor profile for atherosclerosis. Evidence that exercise training consistently improves glycemic control in most patients with type I diabetes is lacking, but improvements in cardiovascular risk factors may nevertheless make regular exercise worthwhile. There is a subgroup of patients with type I diabetes who do well with exercise training. For other patients the goal should be to assist the patient to perform his desired work and recreational activities without major metabolic complications. A great deal of research needs to be done to better outline the specific recommendations for an optimal exercise prescription.

REFERENCES

1. S. Licht, "History," in J. V. Basmajian, Ed., *Therapeutic Exercise,* 4th ed., Williams & Wilkins, Baltimore, 1984, p.3.
2. S. C. S. Sushruta, *Vaidya Jadavaji Trikamji Acharia,* 11/11,12,13,rev. 3rd ed., Nirnyar Sagar Press, Bombay, 1938. The original book was published in 500 B.C.
3. H. Grasset, *La Medicine Naturiste,* Paris, 1911.
4. B. J. Stockvis, *Verhandlungen des Kongresses fur Innere Medizin,* 1886, pp. 126–159.
5. M. Bouchardat, *Annuaire de Therapeutic de Matiere Medical pour 1865,* 1865, pp. 291–336.
6. A. Trousseau, *Glycosuria: Saccharine Diabetes,* Lectures delivered at the Hotel Dieu, Paris, P. Blakiston, Philadelphia, 1882.
7. F. M. Allen, E. Stillman, and R. Fitz, in *Exercise,* Rockefeller Institute, New York, 1916, pp. 486–499.
8. E. Kutz, *Beitrage zur Pathologie and Therapie des Diabetes,* Vol. 1, Marburg, 1874.
9. C. van Noorden, in *Die Zuckerkrankheit und ihre Behandlung,* 2nd ed., Verlag A. Hirschwald, Berlin, 1889, pp. 77–78.
10. J. Rollo, *Cases of Diabetes Mellitus with the Results of the Trials of Certain Acids and Other Substances in the Cure of the Lues Venerea,* 2nd ed., London, 1798.
11. E. P. Joslin, "The Treatment of Diabetes Mellitus," in E. P. Joslin, H. F. Root, P. White, and A. Marble, Eds., *Treatment of Diabetes Mellitus,* Philadelphia, Lea & Febiger, 1959, pp. 243–300.
12. G. Katsch, *Erg. Physikal Diat. Ther.,* **1,** 1 (1939).
13. P. Felig and J. Wahren, *N. Engl. J. Med.,* **293,** 1078 (1975).
14. J. Wahren, *Diabetes,* **28,** Suppl. 1, 82 (1979).
15. G. Ahlborg, P. Felig, L. Hagenfeldt, et al., *J. Clin. Invest.,* **53,** 1080 (1974).
16. S. Maehlum, A. T. Horstmark, and L. Hermansen, *Scand. J. Clin. Lab. Invest.,* **37,** 309 (1977).
17. G. Ahlborg and P. Felig, *Am. J. Physiol.,* **233,** E188 (1977).
18. J. Wahren, P. Felig, and G. Ahlborg, *J. Clin. Invest.,* **50,** 2715 (1971).
19. H. Galbo, N. J. Christensen, and J. J. Host, *Acta Physiol. Scand.,* **101,** 428 (1977).
20. M. Berger, S. Hagg, and N. B. Ruderman, *Biochem. J.,* **146,** 231 (1975).
21. J. Wahren, P. Felig, G. Ahlborg, and L. Jorfeldt, *J. Clin. Invest.,* **50,** 2715 (1971).

22. J. Wahren, L. Hagenfeldt, and P. Felig, *J. Clin. Invest.*, **55,** 1303 (1975).
23. J. Lyngsoe, J. P. Clausen, J. Trap-Jensen, et al., *Clin. Sci. Mol. Med.*, **55,** 73 (1978).
24. L. P. Garetto, E. A. Richter, M. N. Goodman, and N. B. Ruderman, *Am. J. Physiol.*, **246,** E471 (1984).
25. H. Shamoon, R. Hendler, and R. S. Sherwin, *Diabetes,* **29,** 284 (1980).
26. D. H. Wasserman, H. Lavin, A. Lickley, and M. Vranic, *J. Clin. Invest.*, **74,** 1404 (1984).
27. B. Issekutz and M. Vranic, *Am. J. Physiol.*, **238,** E13 (1980).
28. P. F. Blackmore, F. Assimacopoulos-Jeanet, T. M. Chan, and J. H. Exton, *J. Biol. Chem.*, **254,** 2828 (1979).
29. P. Felig and J. Wahren, *J. Clin. Invest.*, **50,** 1702 (1971).
30. B. Issekutz, *Diabetes,* **29,** 629 (1980).
31. N. Altszuler, B. Gottlieb, and J. Hampshire, *Diabetes,* **258,** 116 (1976).
32. A. D. Cherrington, J. L. Chiasson, J. E. Liljenquist, et al., *J. Clinic. Invest.*, **58,** 1407 (1976).
33. H. A. Lickley, G. G. Ross, and M. Vranic, *Am. J. Physiol.*, **236,** E225 (1979).
34. A. E. Roch-Norlund, J. Bergstrom, H. Castenfors, et al., *Acta Med. Scand.*, **187,** 445 (1970).
35. M. Vranic, R. Kawamori, and G. A. Wrenshall, *Diabetes,* **23,** Suppl. 1, 353 (1974).
36. C. A. Sanders, G. E. Levinson, W. H. Abelmann, et al., *N. Engl. J. Med.*, **271,** 220 (1964).
37. P. Felig, O. E. Owen, J. Wahren, et al., *J. Clin. Invest.*, **48,** 584 (1969).
38. W. M. Hunter and M. Y. Sukkar: *J. Physiol. (Lond.),* **196,** 110P (1968).
39. H. Blotner, *Arch. Int. Med.*, **75,** 39 (1945).
40. L. Lutwak and G. Whedon, *Clin. Res.*, **7,** 143 (1959).
41. R. Lipman, P. Raskin, T. Love, et al., *Diabetes,* **21,** 101 (1972).
42. G. Mouratoff and E. Scott, *J.A.M.A.*, **226,** 1345 (1973).
43. H. J. Montoye, W. D. Block, H. Metzner, et al., *Diabetes,* **26,** 172 (1977).
44. B. Saltin, F. Lindgarde, M. Houston, et al., *Diabetes,* **28,** 30 (1978).
45. M. Berger, I. W. Kemmer, K. Becker, et al., *Diabetologia,* **16,** 179 (1979).
46. C. E. Mondon, C. B. Dolkas, and G. M. Reaven, *Am. J. Physiol.*, **239,** 8169 (1980).
47. V. A. Koivisto, V. Soman, P. Conrad, et al., *Am. Soc. Clin. Invest.*, **64,** 1011 (1979).
48. E. A. Nikkila, *Diabtes,* **30,** Suppl. 2, 82 (1981).
49. M. Fahlen, J. Stenberg, and P. Bjorntorp, *Diabetologia,* **8,** 141 (1972).
50. B. Saltin, F. Lingarde, H. Lithell, et al., in W. K. Waldhausl, Ed., *Diabetes,* Int. Cong. Series No. 500, Sept. 1979.
51. P. Bjorntorp, *Adv. Cardiol.*, **18,** 158 (1976).
52. P. Bjorntorp, K. DeJounge, L. Sjostrom, and L. Sullivan, *Metabolism,* **19,** 631 (1970).

53. P. Davidson, S. Shane, and M. Albrink, *Circulation,* **33,** 7 (1966).
54. V. Koivisto, V. Soman, P. Conrad, et al., *J. Clin. Invest.,* **64,** 1011 (1979).
55. M. Vranic and M. Berger, *Diabetes,* **28,** 147 (1979).
56. A. Marble, in A. Marble, P. White, R. Bradley, and L. Krall, Eds., *Joslin's Diabetes Mellitus,* Lea and Febiger, Philadelphia, 1971, p. 291.
57. D. L. Costill, P. Cleary, W. J. Fink, et al., *Diabetes,* **28,** 818 (1979).
58. D. L. Engerbretson, *J. Assoc. Phys. Ment. Rehabil.,* **19,** 74 (1965).
59. H. Wallberg-Henriksson, R. Gunnarsson, J. Henriksson, et al., *Diabetes,* **31,** 1044 (1982).
60. R. A. DeFronzo and N. Kraemer, *Diabetes,* **30,** Suppl. 1, 37 (1981).
61. C. M. Peterson, P. L. Jones, J. A. Esterly, et al., *Diabetes Care,* **3,** 586 (1980).
62. N. B. Ruderman, O. P. Ganda, and K. Johansen, *Diabetes,* **28,** Suppl. 1, 89 (1979).
63. C. Bogardus, E. Ravussin, D. C. Robbins, et al., *Diabetes,* **33,** 311 (1984).
64. D. Caron, P. Poursier, E. B. Marliss, and B. Zinman, *Diabetes Care,* **5,** 364 (1982).
65. J. LeBlanc, A. Nadeau, D. Richard, and A. Tremblay, *Metabolism,* **31,** 453 (1982).
66. J. Gavin, G. Heath, J. Ponser, et al., *Diabetes,* **31,** Suppl. 2, 32A (1982).
67. D. Skor, J. Gavin, J. Hagberg, et al., *Diabetes,* **32,** Suppl. 1, 64A (1983).
68. S. H. Schneider, L. F. Amorosa, A. K. Khachadurian, and N. B. Ruderman, *Diabetologia,* **26,** 355 (1984).
69. M. S. Goldstein, *Am. J. Physiol.,* **20,** 67 (1961).
70. A. Zarzano, T. Balon, L. Garetto, et al., *Am. J. Physiol.,* **248** (1985) (in press).
71. R. J. Jarrett and H. Keen, "Diabetes and Atherosclerosis," in *Complications of Diabetes,* Arnold, London, 1975, pp. 179–203.
72. W. B. Kannel and D. L. McGee, *J.A.M.A.,* 241, 2035 (1979).
73. M. J. Garcia, P. M. McNamara, T. Gordon, and W. B. Kannel, *Diabetes,* **23,** 105 (1974).
74. W. B. Kannel, "Cardiovascular Sequelae of DM," in J. Moskowitz, Ed., *Diabetes and Atherosclerosis Connection,* Juvenile Diabetes Foundation, New York, 1981, pp 5–16.
75. K. W. Beach and D. E. Strandness, *Diabetes,* **29,** 822 (1981).
76. K. M. West, M. M. S. Ahuja, P. H. Bennett, et al., *Diabetes Care,* **6,** 361 (1983).
77. D. W. Strandness, R. W. Priest, and G. E. Gibbons, *Diabetes,* **13,** 336 (1964).
78. F. V. Crall and R. C. Roberts, *Am. J. Med.,* **64,** 221 (1978).
79. C. L. McElroy, S. A. Glissen, and M. C. Fishbein, *Circulation,* **57,** 958 (1978).
80. V. F. Froelicher, *Am. Heart J.,* **84,** 496 (1972).
81. R. W. Eckstein, *Circ. Res.,* **5,** 230 (1957).
82. A. S. Leon and C. M. Bloor, *Circulation,* **41 & 42,** Suppl. 3, 50 (1970).
83. D. M. Kramsch, A. J. Aspen, B. M. Abramowitz, et al., *N. Engl. J. Med.,* **305,** 1483 (1981).
84. J. T. Salonen, P. Puska, and J. Tumilehto, *Am. J. Epidemiol.,* **115,** 526 (1982).

85. T. Ziener-Henriksen, *J. Chronic Dis.*, **29,** 15 (1976).
86. R. S. Paffenbarger, A. L. Wing, R. T. Hyde, et al., *Am. J. Epidemiol.*, **108,** 161 (1978).
87. E. C. Hammond and L. Garfinkel, *Arch. Environ. Health,* **19,** 167 (1969).
88. L. Wilhelmsen, G. Tibblin, M. Aurell, et al., *Adv. Cardiol.*, **18,** 217 (1976).
89. R. Costas Jr., M. R. Garcia-Palmieri, E. Nazario, and P. D. Sorlie, *Am. J. Cardiol.*, **42,** 653 (1978).
90. W. B. Kannel and P. Sorlie, *Arch. Intern. Med.*, **139,** 857 (1979).
91. G. R. Cahill, D. D. Etzwiler, and N. Freinkel, *Diabetes,* **25,** 237 (1976).
92. E. A. Richter, N. B. Ruderman, and S. H. Schneider, *Am. J. Med.*, **70,** 203 (1981).
93. R. Stamler, and J. Stamler, *J. Chronic Dis.*, **32,** 683 (1979).
94. J. Fuller, M. Shipley, G. Rose, et al., *Lancet,* **1,** 1373 (1980).
95. J. L. Witzum, E. M. Mahoney, M. J. Branks, et al., *Diabetes,* **31,** 282 (1982).
96. H. C. Kim, I. Heller, G. Avigad, et al., *Thrombosis and Haemostasis,* **50,** 389 (1983).
97. B. A. McVerry, S. Thorpe, F. Joe, et al., *Haemostasis,* **10,** 261 (1981).
98. R. W. Stout, *Diabetes,* **30,** Suppl. 2, 54 (1981).
99. R. W. Stout, E. L. Bierman, and J. D. Brunzell, "Atherosclerosis and Disorders of Lipid Metabolism in Diabetes, in J. Vallance-Owen, Ed., *Diabetes: Its Physiological and Biochemical Basis,* MTP Press, Lancaster, 1975, pp 125–169.
100. R. W. Stout, *Brit. Med. J.*, **3,** 685 (1970).
101. J. Stamler, R. Pick, and L. N. Katz, *Circ. Res.*, **8,** 572 (1960).
102. N. Peters and C. N. Hales, *Lancet,* **1,** 1144 (1965).
103. E. A. Nikkila, A. A. Miettinen, M. R. Vesenne, and R. Pelkonen, *Lancet,* **2,** 508 (1965).
104. M. Tzagournis, R. Chiles, J. M. Ryan, and T. G. Skillman, *Circulation,* **38,** 1156 (1968).
105. I. Christiansen, T. Deekert, K. Kjerulf, et al., *Acta Med. Scand.*, **184,** 283 (1968).
106. C. Malherbe, M. De Gasparo, P. Berthet, et al., *Eur. J. Clin. Invest.*, **1,** 265 (1970).
107. M. M. Gertler, H. E. Leetma, E. Saluste, et al., *Circulation,* **46,** 103 (1972).
108. L. Kashyap, F. Magill, L. Rojes, and M. M. Hoffman, *Can. Med. Assoc. J.*, **102,** 1165 (1970).
109. F. Sorge, W. Schwartzkopff, and G. A. Neuhaus, *Diabetes,* **25,** 586 (1976).
110. M. M. Gertler, H. E. Leetma, E. Saluste, et al., *Geriatrics,* **27,** 105 (1972).
111. J. M. Sloan, J. S. Mackay, and B. Sheridan, *Diabetologia,* **7,** 431 (1971).
112. T. A. Welborn, A. Breckenridge, A. H. Rubenstein, et al., *Lancet,* **1,** 1336 (1966).
113. R. J. Santen, P. W. Willis, and S. S. Fajans, *Arch. Intern. Med.*, **130,** 833 (1972).
114. K. Pyorala, *Diabetes Care,* **2,** 131 (1979).
115. P. Ducimetiere, L. Schwege, J. L. Papoz, et al., *Diabetologia,* **19,** 205 (1980).
116. T. A. Welborn and K. Wearne, *Diabetes Care,* **2,** 154 (1979).

117. R. Mahler, *Acta Diabetol. Lat.*, **8**, 68 (1971).
118. R. W. Stout, E. L. Bierman, and R. Ross, *Circ. Res.*, **36**, 319 (1975).
119. D. Lohmann, F. Leibold, W. Heilmann, et al., *Metabolism*, **27**, 521 (1978).
120. J. Le Blanc, A. Nadeau, and M. Boulay, *J. Appl. Physiol.*, **46**, 235 (1979).
121. K. Johansen and O. Munck, *Horm. Metab. Res.*, **11**, 424 (1979).
122. J. H. Cuppers, R. Erdmann, H. Schubert, P. Berchtold, and M. Berger, in M. Berger, P. D. Christacopoulos, and J. Wahren, Eds., *Diabetes and Exercise*, Hans Huber, Bern, 1982, p. 155.
123. H. L. Minuk, M. Vranic, E. B. Marliss, et al., *Am. J. Physiol.*, **240**, E458 (1981).
124. A. L. Kennedy, T. R. J. Lappin, T. D. Lavery, et al., *Brit. Med. J.*, **2**, 1191 (1978).
125. G. D. Calvert, J. J. Graham, T. Mannik, et al., *Lancet*, **2**, 66 (1978).
126. B. Michael, M. Camejo, J. Jacobs, et al., *Lancet*, **1**, 155 (1979).
127. M. F. L. Lopes-Virella, P. G. Stone, and J. A. Colwell, *Diabetologia*, **13**, 285 (1977).
128. A. M. Glasgow, G. P. August, and W. Hung, *Diabetes Care*, **4**, 76 (1981).
129. L. Klujber, D. Malnar, M. Kardos, et al., *Eur. J. Pediatr.*, **132**, 289 (1979).
130. B. Dufaux, G. Schimitz, G. Assmann, et al., *Int. J. Sports Med.*, **3**, 58, 123 (1982).
131. C. Diehm, H. Morl, A. Wirth, M. J. Halhuber, G. Schettler, "The Effects of Exercise Training on HDL-Cholesterol in Patients with Coronary Heart Disease," in W. Kindermann and W. Hort, Eds., *Sportmedizin fur Breiten-und Lestungssport*, Demeter Verlag, D-8032 Grafelfing, 1980, pp. 157–162.
132. W. D. Erkelens, J. J. Albers, W. R. Hazzard, et al., *J.A.M.A.*, **242**, 2185 (1979).
133. G. H. Hartung, W. G. Squires, and A. M. Gotto, *Am. Heart J.*, **101**, 181 (1981).
134. M. A. Provost and R. E. Neeves, *Med. Sci. Sports Exerc.*, **13**, 106 (1981).
135. W. D. Erkelens, J. J. Albers, W. R. Hazzard, et al., *Clin. Res.*, **26**, 158 (1978).
136. S. Lopez, R. Vral, L. Balart, et al., *Atherosclerosis*, **20**, 1 (1974).
137. J. O. Holloszy, J. S. Skinner, G. Toro, and T. K. Cureton, *Am. J. Cardiol.*, **14**, 753 (1964).
138. J. K. Huttunen, E. Lansimies, E. Voutilainen, et al., *Circulation*, **60**, 1220 (1979).
139. C. W. Linder, R. H. DuRant, and O. M. Mahoney, *Med. Sci. Sports Exerc.*, **15**, 232 (1983).
140. Z. V. Tran, A. Weltman, G. Glazes, and D. Mood, *Med. Sci. Sports Exerc.*, **15**, 393 (1983).
141. V. P. Steinbrecher and J. L. Witztum, *Diabetes*, **33**, 130 (1984).
142. M. R. Taskinen, E. A. Nikkila, S. Rehunen, and A. Gordin, *Artery*, **6**, 471 (1980).
143. P. D. Thompson, E. Cullinane, L. O. H. Henderson, and P. N. Herbert, *Metabolism*, **29**, 662 (1980).

144. E. Cullinane, S. Siconolfi, A. Saritelli, and P. D. Thompson, *Metabolism,* **31,** 844 (1982).
145. P. D. Wood, W. L. Haskell, S. N. Blair, et al., *Metabolism,* **32,** 31 (1983).
146. G. J. Miller and N. E. Miller, *Lancet,* **1,** 16 (1975).
147. G. G. Rhoads, C. L. Gulbrandsen, and A. Kagan, *N. Engl. J. Med.,* **294,** 293 (1976).
148. D. E. Wilson and R. S. Leers, *J. Clin. Invest.,* **51,** 1051 (1972).
149. A. M. Kapaller-She, *Klincheskaya Med.,* **40,** 79 (1962). Translation in *Fed. Proc.,* **22,** T778 Translation Suppl. (1963).
150. W. Miall and P. Oldham, *Clin. Sci.,* **17,** 400 (1958).
151. H. Montoye, H. Metzner, J. Keller, et al., *Med. Sci. Sports Exerc.,* **4,** 175 (1972).
152. H. L. Taylor, *Can. Med. Assoc. J.,* **96,** 825 (1967).
153. C. B. Thomas, *Ann. Int. Med.,* **53,** 697 (1960).
154. M. Frick and A. Konthinen, *Am. J. Cardiol.,* **12,** 142 (1963).
155. W. Harris, W. Bowerman, P. B. McFadden, and T. A. Kerms, *J.A.M.A.,* **201,** 759 (1967).
156. G. Mann, H. Garrett, A. Farhi, et al., *Am. J. Med.,* **46,** 12 (1969).
157. J. Naughton, K. Shanbour, R. Armstrong, et al., *Arch. Intern. Med.,* **107,** 541 (1966).
158. B. Ekblom, P. Astrand, B. Saltin, et al., *J. Appl. Physiol.,* **24,** 518 (1968).
159. J. Hanson, B. Tabakin, A. Levy, and W. Nedde, *Circulation,* **38,** 783 (1968).
160. M. Rousseau, S. Degre, R. Hessin, et al., *Eur. J. Cardiol.,* **2,** 39 (1974).
161. J. J. Duncan, R. D. Hagan, J. Upton, et al., *Circulation,* **68,** III-285 (1983).
162. P. Bjorntorp, *Hypertension,* **4,** III56 (1982).
163. M. Krotkiewski, K. Mandroukas, L. Sjostrom, et al., *Metabolism,* **28,** 650 (1979).
164. J. A. Colwell, M. G. R. Nair, P. V. Halushka, et al., *Metabolism,* **28,** Suppl. 1, 394 (1979).
165. J. A. Colwell and P. J. Halushka, *Brit. J. Haematol.,* **44,** 521 (1980).
166. R. Ross, *Ann. Rev. Med.,* **30,** 1 (1979).
167. R. Ross, J. Glomset, B. Kariya, et al., *Proc. Natl. Acad. Sci. U.S.A.,* **71,** 1207 (1974).
168. V. Foster, E. Bowie, J. Lewis, et al., *J. Clin. Invest.,* **61,** 722 (1978).
169. T. R. Griggs, R. L. Reddick, D. Sultzer, K. M. Brinkhous, *Am. J. Pathol.,* **102,** 137 (1981).
170. L. Wilhelmsen, K. Suardsudd, K. Korsan-Bengtsen, et al., *N. Engl. J. Med.,* **311,** 501 (1984).
171. J. Kostis, J. Baughman, and P. Kuo, *Chest,* **81,** 571 (1982).
172. I. S. Minon, F. Burke, and H. A. Dewar, *Lancet,* **1,** 700 (1967).
173. R. T. Moxley, P. Brekman, and T. Astrup, *J. Appl. Physiol.,* **28,** 549 (1970).
174. K. Korsan-Bengtsen, L. Wilhelmsen, and G. Tibblin, *Acta Med. Scand.,* **193,** 73 (1973).
175. E. W. Ferguson and M. M. Guest, *Thromb. Diath. Haemorrh.,* **31,** 63 (1974).

176. D. R. Redwood, D. R. Rosing, and S. E. Epstein, *N. Engl. J. Med.*, **286**, 959 (1972).
177. R. S. Williams, E. Logue, J. Lewis, et al., *N. Engl. J. Med.*, **302**, 987 (1980).
178. R. D. Hagan, J. F. Marks, and P. A. Warren, *Diabetes*, **28**, 1114 (1979).
179. O. Olavi, L. Hirvonen, J. Peltonen, and I. Valimak, *Ann. Paediatr. Fenn.*, **11**, 25 (1965).
180. S. Rubler, *N. Y. S. J. Med.*, **81**, 1185 (1981).
181. B. Saltin and L. B. Rowell, *Fed. Proc.*, **39**, 1506 (1980).
182. P. J. Jenkins, R. W. Harper, and P. J. Nestel, *Brit. Med. J.*, **2**, 388 (1978).
183. M. Brownlee and H. Viassara, *Drug Ther.*, March, 66 (1982).
184. T. J. Hahn, S. J. Downing, J. M. Phang, *Am. J. Physiol.*, **220**, 1717 (1971).
185. R. E. H. Wettenhall, P. L. Schwartz, and J. Bornstein, *Diabetes*, **18**, 280 (1969).
186. L. E. Schneider, and H. P. Schedl, *Am. J. Physiol.*, **223**, 1319 (1972).
187. N. S. Ramamurthy, E. J. Zebrowski, C. Baker, et al., *Res. Commun. Chem. Pathol. Pharmacol.*, **5**, 614 (1973).
188. C. A. Hernberg, *Acta Med. Scand.*, **143**, 1 (1952).
189. L. E. Schneider, G. K. Hargis, H. P. Schedl, and G. A. Williams, *Endocrinology*, **95**, 749 (1974).
190. L. E. Schneider, H. D. Wilson, and H. P. Schedl, *Am. J. Physiol.*, **277**, 832 (1974).
191. L. E. Schneider, H. D. Wilson, and H. P. Schedl, *Acta Diabetol.*, **14**, 18 (1977).
192. L. E. Schneider, H. P. Schedl, T. McCain, and M. R. Haussler, *Science*, **196**, 1452 (1977).
193. F. Albright and E. C. Reifenstein, *Parathyroid Glands and Metabolic Bone Disease: Selected Studies*, Williams and Wilkins, Baltimore, 1948, p. 150.
194. J. Menczel, M. Makin, G. Robin, et al., *Isr. J. Med. Sci.*, **8**, 918 (1972).
195. M. E. Levin, V. C. Boisseau, and L. V. Avioli, *N. Engl. J. Med.*, **294**, 241 (1976).
196. J. D. Ringe, F. Kuhlencordt, and J. Kuhnau, Jr., *Dtsch med. Wochenschr.*, **101**, 280 (1976).
197. J. V. Santiago, W. H. McAlister, S. K. Ratzan, et al., *J. Clin. Endocrinol. Metab.*, **45**, 845 (1977).
198. A. L. Rosenbloom, D. C. Lezotte, F. T. Weber, et al., *Diabetes*, **26**, 1052 (1977).
199. J. M. Jurist, *Phys. Med. Biol.*, **15**, 427 (1970).
200. M. D. Klein, H. M. Frost, and E. Sedlin, *Henry Ford Hosp. Med. Bull.*, **12**, 55 (1964).
201. H. M. Frost, *Henry Ford Hosp. Med. Bull.*, **12**, 495 (1964).
202. K. Wu, K. E. Schubeck, H. M. Frost, and A. Villanueva, *Calcif. Tissue Res.*, **6**, 204 (1970).
203. H. E. Meema and S. Meema, *Can. Med. Assoc. J.*, **96**, 132 (1967).
204. H. E. Meema and D. B. W. Reid, *J. Gerontol.*, **24**, 28 (1969).
205. I. DeLeew and R. Abs, *Diabetes*, **26**, 1130 (1977).
206. J. F. Aloia, S. H. Cohn, J. A. Ostuni, et al., *Ann. Int. Med.*, **89**, 356 (1978).

207. B. Krolner, B. Toft, S. Pors Nielsen, and E. Tonderold, *Clin. Sci.*, **64**, 541 (1983).
208. R. A. DeFronzo, R. Hendler, N. J. Christensen, *Diabetes*, **29**, 125 (1980).
209. M. Trovati, Q. Carta, F. Cavalot, et al., *Diabetes Care*, **7**, 327 (1984).
210. V. A. Koivisto and B. Tronier, *Diabetes Care*, **6**, 436 (1983).
211. P. Poussier, B. Zinman, E. B. Marliss, et al., *Diabetes Care*, **6**, 129 (1983).
212. V. A. Koivisto and P. Felig, *N. Engl. J. Med.*, **298**, 77 (1978).
213. P. Dandona, D. Hooke, and J. Bell, *Brit. Med. J.*, **1**, 479 (1978).
214. B. Zinman, F. T. Murray, M. Vranic, et al., *J. Clin. Endocrinol. Metab.*, **45**, 641 (1977).
215. B. Zinman, M. Vranic, A. M. Albisser, et al., *Diabetes*, **28**, Suppl. 1, 76 (1979).
216. M. J. Martin, D. L. Horwitz, M. Nattrass, et al., *Metabolism*, **30**, 688 (1981).
217. M. Vranic and R. Kawamori, *Diabetes*, **28**, 44 (1979).
218. G. Ahlborg and P. Felig, *Am. J. Physiol.*, **233**, E188 (1977).
219. F. W. Kemmer, P. Berchtold, M. Berger, et al., *Diabetes*, **28**, 1131 (1979).
220. R. Kawamori and M. Vranic, *J. Clin. Invest.*, **54**, 331 (1977).
221. D. J. Chisholm, A. B. Jenkins, D. E. James, and E. W. Kraegen, *Diabetes*, **31**, 603 (1982).
222. M. J. Martin, D. C. Robbins, R. Bergenstal, et al., *Diabetologia*, **23**, 337 (1982).
223. A. Schiffrin, S. Parikh, E. B. Marliss, and M. A. Desrosiers, *Diabetes Care*, **7**, 255 (1984).
224. G. Bolli, P. Defeo, P. Compugnacci, et al., *Diabetes*, **32**, 134 (1983).
225. P. E. Cryer and J. E. Gerich, *Diabetes Care*, **6**, 95 (1983).
226. N. H. White, D. A. Skor, P. E. Cryer, et al., *N. Engl. J. Med.*, **308**, 485 (1983).
227. G. Bolli, P. DeFeo, S. DeCosmo, et al., *Diabetes*, **33**, 394 (1984).
228. J. E. Gerich, M. Langlois, C. Noacco, et al., *Science*, **182**, 171 (1973).
229. J. W. Benson, Jr, D. G. Johnson, J. P. Palmer, et al., *J. Clin. Endocrinol. Metab.*, **44**, 459 (1977).
230. J. V. Santiago, W. L. Clarke, S. D. Shah, and P. E. Cryer, *J. Clin. Endocrinol. Metab.*, **51**, 877 (1980).
231. R. M. Bergenstal, K. S. Polonsky, G. Pons, et al., *Diabetes*, **32**, 398 (1983).
232. P. De Feo, G. Bolli, G. Perriello, et al., *Diabetes*, **32**, 887 (1983).
233. M. Ferriere, H. Lachkar, J. L. Richard, et al., *Ann. Int. Med.*, **102**, 134 (1985).
234. S. Ganguli, B. Sterman, P. S. Harris, et al., *Metabolism*, **33**, 845 (1984).
235. M. Berger, P. Berchtold, H. J. Cupper, et al., *Diabetologia*, **13**, 355 (1977).
236. L. Hagenfeldt, *Diabetes*, **28**, Suppl. 1, **66** (1979).
237. H. Dorchy, G. Niset, H. Ooms, et al., *Diabetes Metab.*, **3**, 31 (1977).
238. R. Richardson, *J. Clin. Invest.*, **13**, 949 (1934).
239. W. M. Yater, J. Markowitz, and R. F. Cahoon, *Arch. Intern, Med.*, **51**, 800 (1933).
240. M. J. Whichelow, W. J. H. Butterfield, M. E. Abrams, et al., *Metabolism*, **17**, 84 (1968).

241. M. Williams, E. Gervino, R. Rosa, et al., *Kidney Int.*, **25**, 322 (1984).
242. C. E. Mogensen, C. K. Christensen, and E. Vittinghus, *Diabetes,* **32,** Suppl. 2, 64 (1983).
243. B. F. Waller and W. C. Roberts, *Circulation,* **66,** Suppl. 2, II-283 (1982).
244. M. Silberberg, E. L. Frank, B. S. Jarrett, et al., *Am. J. Pathol.*, **35,** 851 (1959).
245. H. Waine, D. Nevinny, J. Rosenthal, et al., *Tufts Fol. Med.*, **7,** 13 (1961).
246. P. Lee, P. J. Rooney, R. D. Sturrock, et al., *Semin. Arthritis Rheum.*, **3,** 189 (1974).
247. J. Hilsted, H. Galbo, N. J. Christensen, et al., *Diabetologia,* **22,** 318 (1982).
248. W. J. Miller, W. M. Sherman, and J. L. Ivy, *Med. Sci. Sports Exerc.*, **16,** 539 (1984).
249. S. Maehlum and E. D. R. Pruett, *Scan. J. Clin. Lab. Inv.*, **32,** 149 (1973).
250. L. P. Clemow, S. H. Schneider, D. P. Greenfield, et al., *Diabetes,* **33,** Suppl. 1, 27, 7a (1984).

10

Exercise, Diet, and the Rehabilitation of Lung Patients

SUSAN A. GOLDSTEIN, M.S.
and JEFFREY ASKANZI, M.D.

College of Physicians and Surgeons, Columbia University, New York, New York

Malnutrition in hospitalized patients is associated with functional deterioration, including reduced respiratory muscle strength and endurance (1–3) (associated with decreased diaphragmatic mass). Under these conditions a reduction of the ventilatory response to hypoxemia is observed (4). In patients with chronic obstructive pulmonary disease (COPD) the development of malnutrition serves to exacerbate the already existing functional impairments. Unfortunately, weight loss is not only a serious development but also a common occurence in chronic lung disease. As many as 40% of patients diagnosed with COPD experience progressive weight loss, which is associated with a higher rate of mortality (5) in this subgroup. When weight loss develops in a patient with COPD the average life expectancy is only 2.9 years (6). In addition, these patients often become sedentary due to shortness of breath upon exertion.

Supported by Public Health Service Grant HL 23975.

DEFINITIONS

Chronic obstructive pulmonary disease is often categorized into two groups, characterized by the patient's disease state and general appearance. Emphysema patients are considered the "pink puffers," who have hyperinflated lungs and low body weight. Patients with chronic bronchitis are often termed "blue bloaters." The name refers to their tendency to be overweight and to retain carbon dioxide (7). The pink puffers tend to have lung deterioration that corresponds with the degree of nutritional depletion. In addition, they can be futher divided into those with normal levels of arterial CO_2 and CO_2 retainers. It appears that end stage emphysema patients start to develop symptoms that are traditionally associated with chronic bronchitis, such as excessive mucosal secretions and CO_2 retention.

CLINICAL IMPACT AND ETIOLOGY OF WEIGHT LOSS

A number of investigators have observed an association between weight loss and clinical deterioration in patients with COPD. Sukumalchantra and Williams (8) followed 44 COPD patients during a 5 year period and found that the maximal midexpiratory flow rate (MMF) and the lung diffusing capacity (Dco) were reduced in the 12 patients who lost more than 10% of their initial weight. In the 32 patients who had no weight loss, there was no change in the MMF; however, Dco did drop significantly. Results of studies by Vandenbergh and coworkers (5) and Burrows (9) have shown that there is a progressive decline in body weight with advancing pulmonary disease. In addition, this progressive weight loss in COPD patients is associated with negative effects on lung function (10); including an increase in mortality rates (Figure 10-1) and an increased incidence of heart failure compared to those COPD patients without weight loss (1,11,12). Others have shown that weight loss in COPD patients is directly associated with the degree of obstruction to airflow and the severity of the disease (1,11,13).

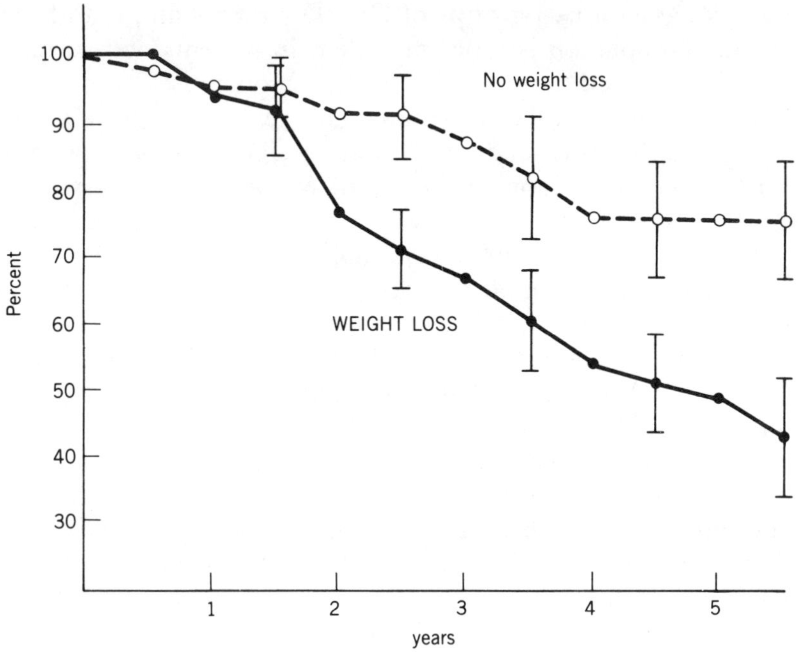

Figure 10-1. Survival rates (mean percentages and standard eror of means) of 114 patients with chronic obstructive pulmonary disease, according to their weight loss.

In malnourished patients without COPD, it has been shown that a severe reduction in body cell mass is associated with significantly lower respiratory muscle strength, specifically a lower peak inspiratory force (P_{Imax})(14). Contrary to popular belief, these studies show that diaphragm weight, respiratory muscle strength, and endurance are reduced in malnourished patients without concomitant clinical signs of pulmonary disease (2,3). In addition, an increased need for mechanical ventilator support has been observed in malnourished patients without COPD (15,16). The respiratory muscles appear to be directly affected by undernutrition. This suggests that malnourished patients with COPD would face even greater demands.

It is apparent that weight loss does not occur in all patients with COPD. Openbrier and coworkers (17) investigated the nutritional status of two groups of COPD patients and found that nutritional depletion is more prevalent in patients with emphysema as compared to those with chronic bronchitis. Patients with emphysema are found to be somatically depleted of protein, and the degree of nutritional depletion is significantly correlated with the degree of lung dysfunction. Many investigators agree that the weight loss in patients with COPD is associated with a marasmic type of protein calorie malnutrition (13,18) involving equal weight loss from all body compartments without a decline in serum albumin.

The cause of the weight loss in patients with COPD is poorly understood. A number of investigators have attributed it to a decrease in caloric intake (1,19). More recently, however, investigators have suggested that an additional cause of weight loss is an increase in the total energy expenditure resulting from the underlying disease process. In malnourished patients with COPD, Hunter and colleagues (13) found that caloric intake was well above predicted energy needs, averaging 2535 cal/day. Other studies, including our own, have supported the concept that weight loss is probably due to an increased resting energy expenditure (REE) (20,21). We have demonstrated that energy expenditure was increased 15% (± 4 SE) prior to nutritional repletion, and 27% (± 4 SE) during the nutritional repletion program. This is unlike the pattern we observe in malnourished surgical patients, who are hypometabolic prior to nutritional repletion with an energy expenditure that equals predicted normal during a nutritional repletion program (1.7 X REE). The increase in resting energy expenditure may be due to an increased work of breathing (Figure 10-2). Since V_E was within normal limits in this group of patients, the increased work of breathing must have been due to a greater load per breath. It has been suggested that weight loss in COPD may be beneficial, since metabolic demands are reduced and this leads to lower ventilatory requirements, alleviating the overworked respiratory muscles. Tiriapur and Afzal (22) have demonstrated that a low calorie, low carbohydrate intake with concomitant weight loss decreases arterial P_{CO_2} and improves respiratory muscle strength

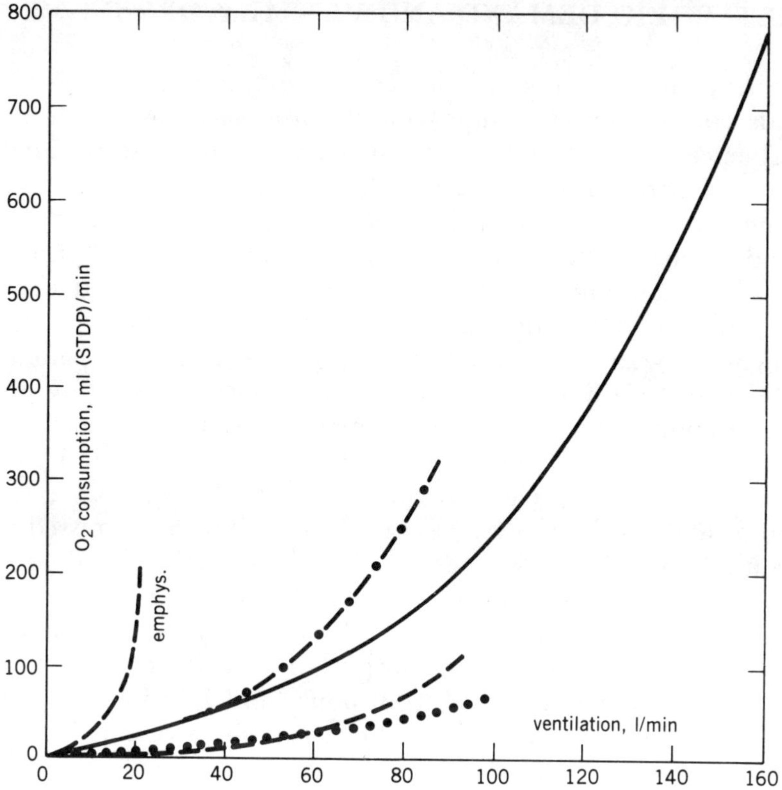

Figure 10-2. Oxygen cost of breathing at various levels of ventilation. The ventilation is increased either by breathing through a dead space or voluntarily (giving CO_2 to avoid hypocapnia). Cournand *et al.* (1954), dead space; Campbell et al. (1957), dead space; Bartlett et al. (1958), voluntary; Milic-Emitli and Petit (1960), dead space, supine.

in overweight hypercapnic patients with COPD. It is clear, however, that this is a different patient population with a less serious clinical picture. In normal weight COPD patients, such as our patient population, weight loss appears to have negative consequences, such as deterioration in respiratory and skeletal muscle strength. Weight loss may be appropriate therapy for overweight patients to alleviate acute physiologic abnormalities, but it is inappropriate for COPD patients of normal body weight.

METABOLIC DEMAND AND VENTILATORY DRIVE

Nutritional intake not only influences lung function by altering body composition and improving defense mechanisms, but also influences respiratory function through alterations in metabolic demand and ventilatory drive. Increasing glucose intake is a stimulus to ventilation, primarily as a result of increased CO_2 production. Carbohydrate is oxidized with a higher respiratory quotient than lipid. Numerous researchers have reported a large rise in CO_2 production with the administration of hypertonic glucose (23–25) which leads to respiratory distress in patients. This is especially true in patients with previously existing lung dysfunction. In malnourished unstressed patients there is a marked rise in CO_2 production when intravenous solutions of glucose and amino acids are administered; the RQ may rise to 1.0 or above if lipogenesis occurs. In malnourished stressed patients, O_2 consumption rises markedly as does CO_2 production, with a more modest rise in the RQ. In either case the rise in CO_2 production will increase the level of ventilation required. Substitution of a fat emulsion for part of the glucose will decrease ventilatory demand (26). Intravenous lipid infusions may decrease the diffusing capacity of O_2 across the alveoli (27); however, this phenomenon has never been observed with an oral fat based diet.

Recent studies have demonstrated that infusion of amino acids results in enhanced ventilatory response to a CO_2 stimulus (28). Normal subjects receiving 5% dextrose followed by intravenous infusion of amino acids demonstrated an enhanced sensitivity to CO_2 during the amino acid infusion. Increasing protein intake to 21g of nitrogen/day with a fixed caloric intake to high levels further enhances the ventilatory response above that observed with a lower nitrogen intake (11 g/day). Increasing glucose intake alone in the absence of amino acids appears to have minimal effects on ventilatory sensitivity (29). Since ventilatory drive may often be markedly increased in many patients with COPD (30), further increases induced by nutritional support may be contraindicated. The COPD patients who received a high carbohydrate diet in the present study had increased ventilation secondary to an increased CO_2 production similar to responses observed in patients without COPD. The effect of amino acid infusions to increase ventilatory drive and the effect of glucose infusions to increase CO_2 production suggest that both protein and glucose must be given in limited quantities. For this reason, a high fat diet might be beneficial for the patient with severe dyspnea or while weaning a patient from mechanical ventilation.

RESPIRATORY AND SKELETAL MUSCLES

It has been demonstrated that respiratory muscle mass and function are compromised in both malnutrition and COPD. The diaphragm, being the principal muscle of respiration, is often used to represent the entire respiratory system. Malnutrition can result in deterioration in both peripheral (31) and respiratory muscle function (32) that exceeds the loss of muscle mass. In addition, malnourished patients undergoing nutritional repletion improve muscle function within 2 weeks, which is long before lean body mass is completely restored. This may indicate that the compromise in muscle function may be due, primarily, to low supply of short-term energy stores or to adverse biochemical alterations of the remaining muscle cells, or both. The changes of muscle function may be due to an increased intracellular calcium concentration found during hypocaloric dieting or to a faulty Na-K ATPase cellular mechanism (33).

Reports indicate that the diaphragm atrophies in malnourished patients (1,34) and may also atrophy in patients with COPD uncomplicated by malnutrition (35). Thus, the combination of malnutrition and COPD may be particularly detrimental (34). Arora and Rochester have shown that patients who are underweight have a reduced diaphragm muscle mass, area, and length independent of the disease state (3). Diaphragm muscle area has been shown to be reduced in patients with COPD (35). These same reports have suggested that there is a significant inverse correlation between diaphragmatic area and the extent of the pulmonary disease in patients with emphysema. However, others have showed that the dimensions of the diaphragm are within normal limits in patients with COPD whose body weight was normal at the time of death (36). In a well-controlled study of elastase-induced emphysema in hamsters, remodeling of diaphragm structure occurred without any effect on mass (36). Chronic increased respiratory workloads in rodents have also been shown to cause histochemical changes in muscle and an increased oxidative capacity of the diaphragm (37). Patients with emphysema and weight loss have a reduced diaphragm weight which exceeds the loss of body weight (4). This is similar to the alterations in diaphragmatic weight observed in malnourished patients without lung disease. Sternocleidomastoid muscle thickness, assessed using anthropomorphic techniques, is reduced in patients with COPD who are of normal weight and even further reduced in COPD patients who have lost weight (38). In summary, it would appear that COPD probably does not cause changes in diaphragmatic weight independent of changes in whole body weight but does cause histological and biochemical adaptations in the diaphragm.

Studies (39,40) have found that respiratory muscle strength is decreased with COPD. In these studies, respiratory muscle strength was measured using maximum static inspiratory and expiratory (P_{Imax}, P_{Emax}) pressures and it was demonstrated that P_{Emax} was uniformly reduced in patients as a function of the severity of the disease. In contrast P_{Emax} was not always reduced in chronic lung disease. This decrease in strength found in patients with COPD may be related to a general weakness of the respiratory muscles. Campbell and coworkers (41) showed that there was a relation between increasing airway obstruction and decreasing amounts of ATP and phosphocreatine (PC) in the intercostal muscles. Other investigators have observed decreased levels of ATP and PC in intercostal and quadriceps muscles in patients with COPD in respiratory distress (42). These low levels of ATP and PC rose in response to nutritional therapy, and concurrently the patient's clinical condition improved.

A decrease in respiratory muscle endurance has also been demonstrated in COPD by measuring maximal voluntary ventilation (MVV)(43,44). In addition, malnutrition has negative effects on MVV in patients without lung disease. Consequently it would be expected that the effects of malnutrition and COPD in combination have a marked negative impact on MVV. In nutritionally depleted patients without COPD, a severe reduction in body cell mass appears to be associated with a reduction in inspiratory muscle strength (14). In patients on mechanical ventilators it appears that nutritional status and supplementation have a major role in determining respiratory muscle strength and the overall clinical condition (15).

TRAINING AND REHABILITATION

Attempts have been made to improve respiratory muscles with exercise based on evidence of increased endurance and strength observed in limb muscles after training (44). It has been shown that COPD patients have a below normal resistance to the development of muscle fatigue during work (43,45). This might be expected because of the lower level of high energy phosphates found in muscles of COPD patients as previously mentioned. Farkas and Roussos (45) have looked at the effect of exercise on the diaphragm in normal hamsters and those with induced emphysema. These investigators found that daily exercise for 1 hour did not influence the diaphragmatic contractile properties in the hamster; however, the development of fatigue was delayed. In addition, hamsters with induced emphysema had a lower degree of diaphragm fatigability. There may be training effect in the respiratory muscles of COPD patients due to the chronic increased work of breathing, and it is felt by these investigators that training the COPD patient may or may not have beneficial effects on the respiratory muscles, since the disease itself results in a form of endurance training on a 24 hour schedule.

There is general agreement that exercise tolerance is improved after training and that the form of exercise, whether it is a treadmill or bicycle, is not important, for as little as 3 weeks of training can show beneficial changes (47–50). Greater improvements have been shown during training programs of longer duration (51,52). The 12 minute walk has been used to test the response to training in the COPD patient. Investigators have shown an increase in the 12 minute walking distance (53,54). Others have focused on training the respiratory muscles with inspiratory resistances in COPD patients with moderate to severe diseases (46,55–58). Measurements included MVV, respiratory muscle strength, and the maximal sustainable ventilatory capacity (MSVC) that could be maintained for 15 minutes under normocapnic conditions. The frequency of training sessions varied between investigators from five times per week to three times daily, 7 days per week. The duration of the session also varied from 5–10 minute bouts to a continuous 30 minute session. The studies showed that training the respiratory muscles improves ventilatory endurance (MVV) (55,58), and respiratory strength (increased resistive load) (57), and increases intensity of ventilation (MSVC) (55,56). However, not all COPD patients were able to benefit from a training program, and therefore either a certain subset of COPD patients may exist that are "unresponsive" or these patients' disease had progressed to a stage that was irreversible. In addition, respiratory muscle training is difficult and the increases in strength and endurance may have small clinical implications (walking performance did not always improve). Also, the long-term benefits are still questionable.

Daily aerobic training at submaximal levels and nonaerobic strength training might be advantageous for these patients as they would result in positive biochemical alterations in the trained muscles and improvement in whole body metabolism. Evidence demonstrates that muscular normal subjects have increased muscle thickness and area, and increased heart weight (59). Any positive effects of training would probably be dependent on the severity of the disease. Respiratory muscle function is also affected by high dose steroids commonly used in chest medicine which are known to cause skeletal muscle wasting leading to respiratory muscle weakness in addition to hypokalemia. Consequently, the overall treatment of the patient must be considered. Finally, the respiratory muscles are also affected by nutritional status. Thus, training during nutritional supplementation of depleted COPD patients may have positive effects on the respiratory muscles; however, this has yet to be determined.

STUDIES IN OUR CLINICAL METABOLIC UNIT

This section will review our clinical experience with refeeding patients with COPD. Preliminary data demonstrating improvement in respiration and skeletal muscle function during nutritional repletion are presented.

Background

An aggressive nutritional support regimen should improve respiratory muscle function but may also increase metabolic demand, thereby increasing the respiratory workload and ultimately causing clinical deterioration. Our goal in designing a nutritional support regimen for patients with lung disease is to provide a diet that will minimize metabolic demands while maximizing functional improvement. In addition, two dietary regimens were studied with the intention of determining the optimal glucose/fat calorie ratio for nutritional supplementation. For this reason the time course of functional improvement during nutritional repletion has been investigated in malnourished patients with COPD.

Previous studies indicated that a 2–3 week feeding regimen is required to affect respiratory muscle function (14,15) in malnourished patients without COPD; thus in the present clinical trials diets were randomly assigned for 1 week each during a 2 to 3 week crossover trial. A thin bore feeding tube was used to provide continuous nasoduodenal feeding which avoided gastric distension and problems such as aspiration associated with either oral or nasogastric feedings. Measurements of metabolic and pulmonary function were performed as were tests of whole body skeletal muscle strength and endurance. We hypothesized that the overall effects of nutritional repletion would be positive and that patients would tolerate the increased metabolic and respiratory demands imposed by nutritional repletion, as a result of improvement in respiratory and peripheral muscle function, if nutritional support was given in modest, measured amounts.

Methods

Patients with a greater than 10% weight loss during the prior year were studied. Six malnourished patients with COPD (forced expiratory volume in seconds/forced vital capacity = 60% predicted) were admitted to the Surgical Metabolic Unit, received enteral nutrition, and were studied for approximately 20 days. One additional patient received parenteral nutrition. All patients were maintained on a stable bronchodilator regimen including theophylline, oral and inhaled beta stimulating drugs, and chest physiotherapy. None of the patients had a history of renal failure, hepatic failure, or diabetes.

The patients received a regular hospital diet for the first 4 days for purposes of acclimatization to the hospital environment and testing procedures. A solution of 5% dextrose (440 kcal/day at 100 ml/hr), plus an appropriate amount of electrolytes, were then infused through a nasoduodenal tube for 36 hours, during which time baseline energy expenditure was measured. Following this period in the first six patients an enteral nutritional support regimen was instituted with a caloric intake of 1.7 × resting energy expenditure (REE). During the period of enteral nutrition two different diets were given for a duration of 6 days each. One diet consisted of 53% carbohydrate, 17% protein, and 30% fat, the other consisted of 28% carbohydrate, 17% protein, and 55% fat; both contained 1.5 kcal/ml solution. The nutritional regimen was provided continuously over a 24 hour period through the nasoduodenal tube throughout the study.

Measurements

Complete blood count (including total lymphocyte count), serum chemistry profile (including albumin), ferritin, iron, and total iron binding capacity were measured weekly. Energy and nitrogen balance were measured continuously on a daily basis to assess changes in fuel utilization. Intake was calculated according to energy and nutritional composition of the enteral diet.

Energy expenditure and ventilatory parameters were measured in supine position using a noninvasive canopy system developed in our laboratory (60,61). Oxygen consumption and CO_2 production were determined 3–5 times each day during 20–30 minute periods evenly spaced throughout the 24 hour period. Ventilatory parameters were measured only on test days. Ventilatory parameters include minute ventilation (V_E), tidal volume (V_T), respiratory frequency (f), inspiratory and expiratory time (T_I, T_E) and inspiratory flow (V_T/T_I). The canopy was ventilated with a continuous airstream of 40 l/min during resting ventilation and was increased to 60 l/min during exercise. The spirometry and gas exchange data were put into the digital computer system and later analyzed. Ventilatory responses during inhalation of 2% and 4% CO_2 were used to assess the ventilatory response to a CO_2 challenge.

Peripheral muscle function was determined as an objective measure of nutritional status, using electrical stimulation to the adductor pollicis muscle (62,63). The test included a force frequency curve, maximal relaxation rate, and maximal voluntary contraction. Ventilatory and metabolic responses to bicycle ergometry in the supine position were performed prior to and weekly following the start of nutritional support. Skeletal muscle strength and endurance were measured in the quadriceps and hamstring muscles using the CYBEX II isokinetic measuring instrument (64). Respiratory muscle function was analyzed according to forced vital capacity (FVC), forced expired volume in one second (FEV_1), peak inspiratory force (PIF), and peak expiratory force (PEF). Measurements were taken prior to nutritional support and weekly thereafter using the methods of Black and Hyatt (65).

Results

The patients we studied had an average weight loss of approximately 14% (Table 10-1). Five of the patients we studied were diagnosed as having emphysema on the basis of clinical history, chest x-ray, decreased diffusion capacity, and an increased residual volume over total lung capacity (RV/TLC), while the first

Table 10-1. Patient Characteristics ($\chi \pm$ SE)

Age	75 ± 3
M^2	1.51 ± .05
% Weight loss	14 ± 1%
Predicted BMR on D_5W	113 ± 5%
Dead space (V_D/V_T)	0.54 ± .05
FVC (% pred)	49 ± 4%
FEV_1 (% pred)	32 ± 5%

patient was diagnosed as a chronic bronchitic based on the same criteria. The age of the patients ranged from 67 to 81 years; their average weight was 46 kilograms. Most patients were limited in daily chores because of shortness of breath. Therefore, isometric bed exercises were encouraged and aerobic exercise was limited to performance tests only. Pulmonary function tests indicate that the patient group had a markedly reduced inspiratory force, vital capacity, and FEV_1. Interestingly the basal metabolic rate in the patients was approximately 13 ± 5% above the predicted value. Energy expenditure rose to 24 ± 4% above predicted after nutritional repletion (caloric intake at 1.7 × REE), as demonstrated in Table 10-2.

The gas exchange and levels of ventilation associated with the

Table 10-2. Energy Expenditure

Subject	D_5W REE Actual/Predicted %	Nutritional Repletion (1.7 × REE) REE Actual/Predicted %
1	−6.2%	18.9
2	14.5%	18.4
3	7.0%	11.5
4	30.4%	35.5
5	15.6%	33.6
6	16.3%	24.5
Average ± SE	13 ± 5%	24 ± 4%

Table 10-3. Changes in Ventilatory Patterns Based on Diet Composition

Rest	D_5W	Cho	Fat
V_E	2.81 ± 0.54	5.28 ± 0.29	4.51 ± 0.34
V_{O2}	136.6 ± 10.9	172.5 ± 11.5	169.6 ± 18.7
V_{CO2}	105.7 ± 6.6	158.1 ± 14.5	135.9 ± 18.7
RQ	.78 ± .04	0.88 ± .05	.80 ± .03
$PaCO_2$	40.5 ± 4.6	41.2 ± 1.7	42.6 ± 2.9
V_T/T_I	205.1 ± 36.5	309.6 ± 31.3	261.4 ± 22.9

two different dietary regimens are shown in Table 10-3. The fat based diet is associated with a similar oxygen consumption and lower CO_2 production than the carbohydrate based diet. The metabolic effects of each regimen were primarily related to macronutrient content. In contrast the functional effects of the diet were unrelated to the composition of the diet but improved with time on either diet in parallel. As shown in Table 10-4 nutritional repletion after 2 weeks resulted in an increase of 11% in quadriceps strength, 37% in hamstring strength, and 44% in leg muscle endurance. However, endurance in these patients was limited because of shortness of breath as opposed to skeletal muscle fatigue. Thus, the results indicate an improved respiratory en-

Table 10-4. Effects of Refeeding: % Change in Skeletal and Respiratory Muscle Function (χ ± SE)

	Week 2	Week 3
Quadriceps strength	11 ± 7	44 ± 19[a]
Hamstring strength	37 ± 11[a]	65 ± 18[a]
Endurance/power[b]	44 ± 12[a]	46 ± 17[a]
Forced vital capacity	16 ± 10	24 ± 7[a]
Forced expiratory volume	18 ± 9	21 ± 6[a]

[a](p .05)
[b]Endurance times strength.

durance. In the patients studied for a third week a further improvement was observed. The respiratory muscles showed a 24 $\pm$ 7% improvement in FVC and a 21 $\pm$ 6% improvement in FEV_1 during hospitalization (p .05).

These results demonstrate a number of important phenomena that could be helpful in the treatment of chronic obstructive lung disease. It is clear that nutritional repletion can be safely given to nutritionally depleted patients with chronic obstructive pulmonary disease at the start of their weight loss. Also, refeeding significantly improves overall function and has a positive effect on body composition: an increase in lean body mass with a concomitant diureses. However, there did not seem to be dramatic improvement in the patient studied with advanced disease and cor pulmonale. Exercise was not possible and caloric intake was very limited as a result of severe shortness of breath. No significant beneficial changes occurred. Another patient with severe COPD and cor pulmonale was unable to tolerate a caloric intake above REE and was eventually dropped from the program. If this finding is confirmed in other similar patients it would indicate that our ability to improve the condition of such patients is far more limited than it is in those patients with emphysema alone and that refeeding must begin at the start of weight loss. This is probably related to a greater loss in respiratory muscle strength along with water retention which occurs in end stage of COPD with cor pulmonale.

Nutritional therapy appears to have an increasingly important role in malnourished patients with COPD based on evidence of an increased energy expenditure, and the influence of macronutrients on ventilation. Thus, it is advisable that COPD patients initiate a high caloric intake at the first signs of unaccountable weight loss. Meals should consist of six small feedings to minimize metabolic demands and a high fat diet is advisable during episodes of respiratory distress to maximize the ratio of oxygen consumption to minute ventilation. In addition, evidence suggests that submaximal aerobic training and isometric exercises may improve respiratory and skeletal muscles, and produce an overall feeling of well being.

In conclusion, the weight loss in COPD is associated with hypermetabolism, and caloric intake may not be sufficient to meet increased metabolic demands, thereby contributing further to this progressive and inexplicable weight loss. This is in contrast to depleted surgical patients, who have energy expenditures 5% below predicted. There is an increased minute ventilation in patients receiving a high carbohydrate diet, secondary to an increased VCO_2, which is similar to that seen in patients with neither COPD nor weight loss. Ventilatory drive appears to be influenced by nutritional repletion. Respiratory and skeletal muscle function increase, particularly strength, endurance, and work efficiency, indicating that the increased metabolic demand can be well tolerated.

REFERENCES

1. W. M. Thurlbeck, *Thorax*, **33**, 483 (1978).
2. N. S. Arora and D. F. Rochester, *Am. Rev. Respir. Dis.*, **126**, 5 (1982).
3. N. S. Arora and D. F. Rochester, *J. Appl. Physiol.*, **52**, 64 (1982).
4. H. Baier and P. Somani, *Chest*, **85**, 222 (1984).
5. E. Vandenbergh, K. P. Van de Woestijne, and A. Gyselen *Am. Rev. Resp. Dis.* **95**, 556 (1967).
6. E. Vandenbergh, K. P. Van de Woestijne, L. Billiet, and A. Gyselen, *Bull. Physiopath. Resp.*, **1**, 260 (1965).
7. A. C. Dornhorst, *Lancet*, **1**, 1185 (1955).
8. Y. Sukumalchantra and M. H. Williams, *Am. J. Med.*, **39**, 441 (1965).
9. B. A. Burrows, A. H. Nidon, W. R. Barclay, and J. E. Kasik, *Am. Rev. Respir. Dis.*, **91**, 665 (1964).
10. A. G. Driver, M. T. McAlevy, and J. L. Smith, *Chest*, **82**, 568 (1982).
11. A. D. Renzetti, D. H. McClement, and B. D. Litt, *Am. J. Med.*, **41**, 115 (1966).
12. S. F. Boushy, P. K. Adhikair, A. Sakamota, et al., *Dis. Chest*, **45**, 402 (1964).
13. A. M. B. Hunter, M. A. Carey, and H. W. Larsh, *Am. Rev. Resp. Dis.*, **124**, 376 (1981).
14. S. M. Kelly, A. Rosa, S. Field, et al., *Am. Rev. Respir. Dis.*, **130**, 33 (1984).
15. H. R. Bassili and M. Dietel, *J.P.E.N.*, **5**, 161 (1981).
16. A. G. Driver and M. LeBrun, *J.A.M.A.*, **244**, 2195 (1980).
17. D. R. Openbrier, M. M. Irwin, R. M. Rogers, et al., *Chest*, **88**, 17 (1983).
18. R. M. Rogers, J. H. Dauber, M. H. Saunder, et al., *Chest*, **85**, 635 (1984).
19. N. L. Wilson, R. H. L. Wilson, and S. M. Farber, *J. Am. Diet. Assoc.*, **45**, 530 (1964).

20. D. R. Openbrier, M. M. Irwin, J. H. Dauber, et al., *Chest*, **85**, 675 (1984).
21. S. P. Heymsfield, A. Head, G. Grossman, and G. W. Stanton, *J.P.E.N.*, **5**, 562 (1981).
22. V. Tiriapur and M. Afzal, *Am. J. Med.*, **77**, 987 (1984).
23. J. Askanazi, D. H. Elwyn, P. A. Silverberg, et al., *Surgery*, **87**, 596 (1980).
24. H. D. Covelli, J. W. Black, M. V. Olsen, and J. F. Beekman, *Ann. Int. Med.*, **95**, 579 (1981).
25. T. Gieseke, G. Gurushanthaiah, and F. L. Glauser, *Chest*, **71**, 55 (1977).
26. J. Askanazi, J. Nordenstrom, S. H. Rosenbaum, et al., *Anesthesiology*, **54**, 373 (1981).
27. R. F. Inwood, P. Gora, and C. E. Hunt, *Prostagland. Med.*, **6**, 503 (1981).
28. J. Askanazi, C. Weissman, P. Lasala, et al., *Anesthesiology*, **60**, 106 (1984).
29. J. Rodriguez, C. Weissman, J. Askanazi, et al., *J.P.E.N.*, **5**, 573 (1982).
30. J. Milic-Emili, *Lung*, **160**, 1 (1982).
31. J. Lopes, D. M. Russell, J. Witwell, et al., *Am. J. Clin. Nut.*, **36**, 602 (1982).
32. I. M. Fraser, D. McK. Russel, S. Whittaker, et al., *Am. Rev. Resp. Dis.*, **129**, A269 (1984).
33. D. M. Russell, P. M. Walker, L. A. Leiter, et al., *Am. J. Clin. Nut.*, **39**, 503 (1984).
34. C. Butler, *Am. Rev. Respir. Dis.*, **114**, 155 (1976).
35. N. S. Arora and D. F. Rochester, *Am. Rev. Respir. Dis.*, **123**, 176 (1982).
36. S. G. Kelson, T. Wolanski, G. S. Supinskli, and U. Roessman, *Am. Rev. Respir. Dis.*, **129**, 330 (1983).
37. T. G. Keens, V. Chen, P. Patel, et al., *J. Appl. Physiol.*, **44**, 905 (1978).
38. N. S. Arora and D. F. Rochester, *Chest*, **85**(Suppl.), 588 (1984).
39. N. M. T. Braun and D. F. Rochester, *Am. Rev. Resp. Dis.*, **117**, 91 (1979).
40. D. F. Rochester, N. S. Arora, N. M. T. Braun, et al., *Bull. Physiopathol. Respir.*, **15**, 951 (1979).
41. T. J. H. Clark, S. Freedman, E. J. M. Campbell, et al., *Clin. Sci.*, **36**, 307 (1969).
42. T. K. Aldrich, N. S. Arora, and D. F. Rochester, *Am. Rev. Respir. Dis.*, **126**, 195 (1982).
43. J. A. Campbell, R. L. Hughes, V. Sahgal, et al., *Am. Rev. Respir. Dis.*, **122**, 697 (1980).
44. I. Gertz, G. Hedenstierna, G. Hellers, and J. Wahren, *Clin. Sci. Molec. Med.*, **52**, 395 (1977).
45. G. A. Farkas and C. Roussos, J. Appl. Physiol. Respir. Environ. Exercise. Physiol.
46. R. L. Pardy, R. N. Rivington, and P. J. Despas, *Am. Rev. Respir. Dis.*, **123**, 426 (1981).
47. T. L. Petty, L. M. Nett, M. M. Fenegan, et al., *Ann. Intern. Med.*, **70**, 1109 (1969).
48. J. E. Hodgkin, "Pulmonary Rehabilitation," in D. H. Simmons, Ed., *Current Pulmonology*, Vol. 3, Wiley, New York, 1981, pp. 361-380.

49. M. M. Lertzman and R. M. Chernack, *Am. Rev. Respir. Dis.*, **114,** 1145 (1976).
50. K. M. Moser G. C. Bokinsky, R. J. Savage, et al. *Arch. Intern. Med.*, **140,** 1596 (1980).
51. O. J. Mertens, R. J. Shepherd, and T. Kavanaugh, *Respiration*, **34,** 96 (1978).
52. J. J. Nicholas, R. Gilbert, R. Gave, et al., *Am. Rev. Respir. Dis.*, **102,** 1 (1978).
53. D. J. M. Sinclair and C. G. Ingram, *Brit. Med. J.*, **1,** 519 (1980).
54. A. E. Brockcroft, M. J. Sanders, and G. Berry, *Thorax*, **36,** 200 (1981).
55. L. Peress, P. McClean, C. Woolf, and N. Zamel, *Am. Rev. Respir. Dis.*, **119,** 157 (1979).
56. M. J. Belman and C. Mittman, *Am. Rev. Respir. Dis.,* **121,** 273 (1980).
57. J. B. Andersen, L. Dragsted, T. Kann, et al., *Scand. J. Respir. Dis.*, **60,** 151 (1979).
58. L. J. Sonne and J. A. Davis, *Chest*, **81,** 436 (1982).
59. D. F. Rochester, unpublished data, March, 1985.
60. J. M. Kinney, A. P. Morgan, F. J. Dominguez, and K. J. Gildner, *Metabolism*, **13,** 205 (1964).
61. J. L. Spencer, B. A. Zikria, J. M. Kinney, et al., *J. Appl. Physiol.,* **33,** 523 (1972).
62. P. A. Merton, *J. Physiol.*, **123,** 553 (1954).
63. R. H. T. Edwards, A. Young, G. P. Hosking, and D. A. Jones, *Clin. Sci. Mol. Med.*, **52,** 283 (1977).
64. D. A. Murray, E. Harison, and G. A. Wood, Med Sci. Sports Exerc. **14,** 177 (1982).
65. L. F. Black and R. E. Hyatt, *Am. Rev. Resp. Dis.*, **99,** 696 (1969).

11

Interrelations of Exercise and Diet on Bone Metabolism and Osteoporosis

MORRIS NOTELOVITZ, M.D., Ph.D.

University of Florida, Gainesville, Florida

Osteoporosis is a condition that cripples millions of women with chronic and psychologic pain; women who once stood erect have to face daily life as bent "little old ladies" and suffer the indignity of not even being able to purchase a garment that fits their misshapen bodies. Osteoporosis is also a condition that can cause premature death. Each year over 300,000 women in the United States will fracture their hips as a result of osteoporosis. Approximately 10 to 15% will die within 6 months of complications resulting from this event (1), while only about one-third of women will ever return to a rehabilitated normal life (2). Yet, despite the severity of this condition and its complex multifactorial etiology, osteoporosis can, in all probability, be prevented by the simple expedients of appropriate exercise and good nutrition. Central to the issue is the fact that bone is a living organ.

THE BONE REMODELING CYCLE

Bone formation is dependent on a five-stage cycle that results in old bone being removed and replaced with new bone. Normally, this process is coupled; the amount of old bone removed is replaced with an equal amount of freshly formed bone. Initiation of the cycle is dependent on the recruitment and activation of osteoclasts. This activity usually takes place on the inner aspect of the bone's surface—the endosteal layer—and results in the dissolution of bone mineral and collagen, and the formation of a cavity. Resorption ceases when the mean depth of the cavity reaches 60 μm (trabecular bone) to 100 μm (cortical bone) from the surface (3). At this point, mononuclear cells lay down a highly mineralized collagen-poor bone matrix known as cement substance. It is from this surface that new bone is laid down by osteoblasts (4). These cells probably originate from bone marrow stromal stem cells (preosteoblasts), thereby sharing the ability of another cell type, the fibroblast, to synthesize collagen (5). The stimulus to osteoblast recruitments may be mechanical or due to humeral or locally produced substances; for example, human skeletal growth and other bone growth factors (6).

The osteoblasts are responsible for the synthesis of collagen, which is the main component of newly formed bone matrix, or osteoid. The latter matures and is later mineralized by a process that is largely dependent on an adequate supply of calcium and phosphate and the formation of hydroxyapatite crystals (3). At a microstructural level, numerous small crystallites of hydroxyapatite may be seen in intimate juxtaposition and in a highly organized geometric arrangement with collagen fibrils (7).

The elastic and tensile strength of bone is dependent in large measure on this combined interrelationship. Another very important determinant of the mechanical strength of bone is the orientation of the collagen fibrils in the bone matrix and the three-dimensional network of plates and bars found especially in trabecular bone (for example, in vertebrae), and to a lesser extent in cortical bone (for example, the radius). This results in a scaffold-like arrangement of vertical and horizontal trabeculae. Interruption of this support system, for example, loss of horizontal trabeculae due to ageing, can impair the structural integrity of the bone and result in fracture, even in the presence of a relatively normal amount of bone mineral.

TYPES AND RATES OF BONE LOSS

There are two types of bone: cortical and trabecular. Cortical (compact) bone is found primarily in the appendicular skeleton, for example, in the femur, tibia, and fibula of the lower limbs and the humerus, ulna, and radius of the arms. Cortical bone constitutes 80% of the total skeleton but is metabolically less active than trabecular bone. About 10% of the cortical bone is remodeled each year. Trabecular (cancellous) bone is found in the axial skeleton, primarily in the vertebral bodies (70–95%), with lesser concentrations in areas such as the neck of the femur (25–35%) and the distal radius (5–20%). The remodeling process is far more active in trabecular bone partly because the architectural arrangement of the bone plates provides a larger exposed surface area for exchange with the extracellular compartment. Approximately 40% of trabecular bone is remodeled each year. It is because of this greater activity that vertebral osteoporosis occurs more frequently.

After longitudinal bone growth has been achieved, further increase in the bone mineral content and mass of bone occurs until about age 35, at which point the individual is said to have achieved maximal cortical bone mass. From this age until the onset of menopause, it is normal for women to lose about 0.12% of the cortical bone per year; after the menopause and until age 65, the rate of bone loss increases to about 1% per year, slowing down after 65 to 0.18% per year. This physiologic bone loss averages out to a 25% decrease in cortical bone mass over a 30 year age span—from 50 to 80 years (8). Trabecular bone accrual reaches its maximal mass during the mid- to late twenties, and is followed thereafter by a linear loss of bone (9). Others maintain that the trabecular bone loss pattern is equal to that of the cortical bone, with a 0.19% loss per year before the menopause, and a 1.1% loss thereafter. It has been estimated that 31.7% of trabecular bone is lost during the 50 year span between 30 and 80 years of age (8).

Bone loss occurs either because the osteoclasts erode cavities that are too deep or because osteoblasts lay down insufficient bone. The latter process is said to account for the slow loss of bone associated with aging and the former with a rapid bone loss that can actually result in focal perforation of the trabecular plates, with a resultant loss in the continuity and, hence, mechanical support. The two mechanisms may function in concert and account for the abrupt increase in vertebral fracture rate that sometimes follows estrogen withdrawal or conditions where the bone mass is already reduced; for example, in patients with hyperthyroidism. A similar process of increased subendosteal porosity is also said to weaken cortical bone (10); increased longitudinal tunneling occurs with an increase in bone remodeling without necessarily an excessive loss of bone mineral. At this time, it is not possible to clinically evaluate the degree of microdamage that may be present, and reliance has to be placed on the presence of overt, radiologically apparent fractures. This has resulted in the differentiation of osteopenia (decreased bone mineral content without fractures) from osteoporosis (decreased bone mass with identifiable fractures).

Osteopenia is potentially reversible; osteoporosis is irreversible in the sense that the distorted bone architecture of a fractured vertebra cannot be restored to normal. Prevention of osteoporosis depends largely upon the accrual of as much bone as possible before the menopause. Simply stated, the more bone an individual has, the more she can afford to lose without impairing the skeleton's strength.

EXERCISE, BONE MASS, AND STRENGTH

It has long been recognized that mechanical force plays an important role in bone formation and function. This is especially true for cortical bone. What is not known, however, is how much exercise is needed and whether there is an optimal form of exercise for bone accrual.

The structural and mechanical demands of the skeleton vary. Whereas the skull bone experiences very little stress during normal daily activity, the lower extremities are exposed to thousands of loading and unloading cycles per day. A given amount of activity is necessary to maintain a level of normal bone mass. It is postulated (11) that there is a physiologic band of activity that is site-specific: immobilization can lead to severe bone loss at some sites while repeated loading at high strain magnitudes can result in bone hypertrophy. Further, the frequency and degree of activity may be critical. Repeated and prolonged exercise can cause bone fatigue and microscopic damage. If this microdamage occurs at a slow rate, normal bone turnover will repair the microfractures, maintain the structural integrity, and maybe result in hypertrophy of the bone; repeated or excessive strain applied to areas of microdamage will stimulate increased bone tissue removal by osteoclasts and, by an accumulation of damage, result in a weakening of the bone, and stress factors commonly associated with prolonged exercise, such as long distance running.

The bone's response to exercise is also age and strain related. Based on animal data, it is suggested that bone mass accrual is much more responsive to a given mechanical strain in growing than in mature bone. This underlines the importance of encouraging young women to exercise in preparation for the anticipated postmenopausal bone loss. Both animal experimentation and clinical experiences have shown that the accumulation of appropriate mechanical damage can serve as a stimulus to bone hypertrophy. This will require the exposure of adult bone to cyclic strain levels of 2000 microstrain or more. However, there is an optimum level above which increasing strain levels will not enhance bone mass and may even have a negative effect.

It is important to differentiate the amount of exercise needed to maintain bone mass from that which may result in bone hypertrophy. Bone mineral is lost with simple bed rest. Depending on the method of bone mass measurement used, variable rates of bone loss have been reported; the average rate appears to be 4% per month during the initial phase of bed rest (12). When hypercalciuria is used as a measure of lost bone mineral, the peak loss appears to occur at about 7 weeks and reaches a steady state by 25 weeks. Prolonged bed rest can cause a negative calcium balance of 200–300 mg/day. It has also been noted that subjects with higher initial bone mass lose bone more than those with lower values; eventually all immobilized patients seem to end up with a similar bone mass (12). Trabecular bone appears to be more sensitive to cessation of mechanical loading than cortical bone (13). Gravity, per se, plays an important role; weightlessness in space results in a long-term reduction of the bone mineral content (−5% in the os calcis) commensurate with the duration of the loss of gravity (14). In determining the amount of weight-bearing needed to prevent this bone loss, it was found that 3 hours a day of quiet standing had a partial effect, while 4 hours of walking could prevent bone loss associated with 20 hours of bed rest (15). Isometric or horizontal exercise in bed is not able to restore the bone loss associated with immobilization.

A number of clinical studies have been published that attest to the benefit of exercise. Thus, athletes (16), cross-country runners (17), ballet dancers, and weight lifters (18), all have higher than average bone mass. Bone mass accrual is related to the type of exercise performed; the higher levels of bone mineral in the distal femur of weight lifters, runners, and soccer players, for example, is not found in swimmers (16). Similarly, male marathon runners do not have a higher midshaft radius bone mineral content, but they do have a significantly higher total body calcium content.

Prospective studies have confirmed the bone-building potential of exercise in both men and women (19–22). Different exercise regimens have been reported but what is lacking is a definitive guide to the type and amount of exercise needed to improve bone mass. The study by Jones and coworkers illustrates that exercise may have both systemic effects and a local effect. Professional tennis players were found to have an overall greater bone mass than age-matched casual tennis players, but in addition, the cortical thickness of the playing arm in the professional players was 34.9% greater than in their nonplaying (control) arm. The same was found in female professionals; the cortical thickness in the dominant arm was 28.4% greater than in their (control) nondominant arm.

In attempting to derive a prescription of optimum exercise for the prevention of osteoporosis, two animal studies may provide the direction needed. In a series of experiments, Lanyon (23) recently summarized certain principles that could maximally benefit bone remodeling through exericse. Three main points emerge:

1. To overcome the potential bone atrophy, a minimum peakstrain of 1000 microstrain is necessary to maintain normal bone formation. Strains (load-bearing) above this level were associated with a proportional increase in new bone formation. The clinical message: low strain levels may maintain the bone's structural status by preventing bone resorption; high strain levels are needed for osteogenesis.

2. Relatively few strain cycles are needed to influence positively the bone remodeling cycle. By applying as few as 36 consecutive 0.5 Hz load cycles per day, the bone mineral content at the midshaft of an adult rooster's ulna was increased by 33% over a 6 week period. No additional new bone formation resulted from increasing the number of repetitions to 360 or 1800 cycles per day. Therefore, exercise designed to hypertrophy bone does not have to be repeated often. To prevent resorptive remodeling and a decline in bone mass, only four cycles of a similar load regimen were needed. In all probability, everyday activity will be sufficient to maintain normal bone mass.

3. The functional stimulus to bone remodeling must be dynamic. Static (compressive) force may have a negative influence. Strain levels imposed at fast physiologic rates will stimulate an increase in bone mass, whereas similar levels at slow strain rates may be associated with resorption. In short, for an exercise regimen to be osteogenic, it should be diverse and vigorous. Since the maximum effect is achieved rapidly, the exercise need not be repeated often.

A further guide is derived from the distribution of porosity in long bones and highlights engineering rather than medical principles (23a). Most of the intracortical loss in long bones is in the anterior and posterior compartments, areas that are less frequently exposed to stress. Mechanical force applied to long bones results in lateral bending. The resultant compressive force generated on the medial side and the tensile force on the lateral aspect of the bone results in osteogenesis, and, hence, greater mechanical strength in the area of the bone needed for greatest support.

In this context, muscle strengthening/resistant exercises, for example, the use of nautilus exercise equipment, should provide the optimum approach to achieving bone hypertrophy. The technique allows for rapid repetitions of appropriately distributed mechanical strain to be applied to specific regions of the skeleton for short periods.

The success of any exercise program will depend on the individual's motivation and compliance, and therefore, enjoyment of a given exercise. A program that will simultaneously improve cardiovascular fitness would be an added incentive and advantage, since cardiovascular-related disease is the major cause of death in postmenopausal women. The study of Woo and coworkers (24) provides some insight into the potential value of running as a stimulus to new bone formation. They exercised 1 year old pigs for 60 minutes/day, at a rate that was equivalent to 65 to 80% of their maximum heart rate. When compared with nonexercised controls, a 17% increase in cortical thickness was recorded, as well as an increase in bone strength. The bone density and biochemical content of the control and exercised animals were the same.

Thus, prolonged aerobic exercise in animals has been found to have a significant effect on the quantity, but not the quality of bone. By extrapolation, the author suggested that exercise comparable to that prescribed in running fitness programs for humans (65–80% of maximum heart rate) would not only maintain bone homeostasis, but could produce bone hypertrophy. Emiola and O'Shea (25) determined that young adults (20 to 25 years of age) required at least 3 hours of moderate activity to increase bone density.

The qualitative, rather than the quantitative improvement in bone strength resulting from aerobic exercise may be due to yet another engineering principle—an increase in bone width. Radial expansion of long bones is an important determinant of bone strength. The so-called cross-sectional moment of inertia (CSMI) is what determines the resistance of bone to bending. Increase in the external diameter of the bone—brought about by increased periosteal (outer layer) new bone formation—can compensate for the inevitable loss in the quality of bone tissue that occurs with ageing. The improvement in the CSMI in men, is said to be a major reason why they do not suffer long bone fractures to the same extent as age-matched females (25).

Can you exercise too much? Young rats run on a 5 degree inclined treadmill at 30 cm/second for 30 minutes a day (moderate training) were found to increase the femural bone weight. When training was extended to 180 minutes per day, the femural bone volume and length decreased (26). Women marathon runners, whose activity was associated with exercise-induced amenorrhea, were noted to have a reduced amount of trabecular bone in their lumbar vertebrae (as measured by dual photon absorptiometry), with normal or minimally reduced cortical bone (as measured by single photon absorptiometry and radiogrammetry) (27,28). The reason for this bone loss has been attributed to estrogen deficiency (associated with decreased body fat) and hyperprolactinemia (28).

A group of women who ran a similar distance each week (40 miles) but who were still menstruating, had a significantly greater bone mineral content at the midshaft and distal shaft of the radius when compared with a matched control group (29), but a significantly lower density of the os calcis (mainly trabecular bone). By retaining their menstrual function (and, presumably, normal ovarian steroidgenesis) these women were able to increase their cortical bone mass, but as with other long-distance runners, had lower trabecular bone values. It is important to differentiate between changes brought about by exercise-induced (intense) amenorrhea and appropriate exercise in women with preexisting amenorrhea. Women with anorexia nervosa—all of whom were amenorrheic and hypoestrogenic—and who were physically active, had significantly greater bone mass than a similar group of inactive anorectics (30). It would appear that moderate exercise in women is osteogenic, even in the presence of an estrogen deficiency state; that one may be able to stimulate cortical bone hypertrophy in women with intact ovarian function by intense activity, but that this may occur at the expense of the trabecular component of the skeleton.

The mechanism whereby exercise stimulates new bone formation is not clearly established. Mechanical load, muscular activity, and gravity serve as an extracellular stimulus that is transmitted to bone cells to initiate their genetic program for growth and differentiation. Intermediaries include events such as the generation of piezoelectricity that stimulates cyclic-nucleotide activity, prostaglandin synthesis, and other matrix-derived bone growth factors (6,31,32). What has been established, however, is that exercise is directly associated with the laying down of matrix on the remodeling surfaces of the bone's trabeculae and cortices. The matrix is composed primarily of collagen. Chvapil and coworkers (33) showed that the amount and concentration of collagen in the femora of adult rats increased with exercise but that no effect on the calcium content occurred. This experiment serves to illustrate a most important point: to benefit from exercise and its osteogenic stimulus, it is necessary to ensure an adequate supply of the substrate (mainly, calcium) needed to mineralize and mature the newly formed bone. It is well known that fluoride therapy without simultaneous calcium supplementation will increase mineralization of the axial skeleton, but at the expense of the cortical bone and an increase in hip fractures (34). A similar situation may be true for exercise-induced osteogenesis, except in this instance it is the cortical bone that benefits at the expense of the trabecular compartment. This may prove to be one of the reasons that the amenorrheic woman reported by Drinkwater and coworkers (27) had lower spiral, but not cortical, bone mineral when compared with the eumenorrheic controls. Although both groups met the current recommended dietary allowance of 800 mg of elemental calcium per day, the amenorrheic subjects fell short of the recommended amount needed to maintain calcium balance in low estrogen states (1500 mg of elemental calcium per day) whereas the eumenorrheic women met this daily requirement (27).

Exercise in women with established osteoporosis has to be modulated by the fact that preexisting microfractures and discontinuity between the trabecular plates, especially in the axial skeleton, could be aggravated by weight-bearing exercise. Furthermore, even though individual fragments of the horizontal trabecular plates may be hypertrophied by exercise, the loss of their continuity, and hence, structural integrity, will still deprive the bone from improving in strength and in response to stress. Nevertheless, light to moderate exercise in older women has resulted in an improvement of the cortical bone mass. Smith and coworkers (20) designed an exercise program for elderly women (mean age, 81) that oriented activity (1.5 to 3.0 METS in intensity) around a chair. One MET equals a maximal oxygen uptake of 3.5 ml/minute/kg, which is the average value of effort obtained on subjects during chair rest. Over a 3 year period, their exercise group demonstrated a 2.29% increase in midshaft radius bone mineral content, whereas a matched control group lost 3.29% of their bone mineral content. Walking is the safest and most effective form of exercise for women with osteoporosis.

DIET AND BONE HEALTH

In fully mature bone the protein matrix—consisting in the main of collagen embedded in a mucopolysaccharide ground substance—accounts for 35% of the volume of the intercellular material, with mineral occupying most of the remainder. The hydroxyapatite crystal in mineralized bone contains significant amounts of sodium, magnesium, carbonate, and citrate iron, but calcium and phosphorus are the principal minerals. Factors that regulate their supply, absorption, deposition, and withdrawal from bone, underly the importance of nutrition and its role in maintaining bone health.

Calcium

Absorption and Needs. The amount of calcium in blood, in extracellular fluid, and in the extraosseous cellular compartments accounts for 1% of the total body calcium. The calcium in bone is available to the circulation through an established but ill-understood mechanism involving a pool of readily exhange-able soluble bone calcium. This pool serves as an immediate reservoir for plasma calcium to ensure that a steady state is maintained and to meet the need for calcium in processes as diverse as coagulation of the blood, nerve transmission, cardiac function, and muscle contraction.

Skeletal growth during childhood requires the retention of 150 mg of calcium per day; adolescence and early adulthood, when bone growth is maximal, results in 275 to 500 mg of calcium per day being deposited in bone. During later adult life, when bone growth is replaced by bone maintenance, less calcium is required, but still averages 180 g per year. Translated into recommended daily allowances of calcium, infants [less than 1 year] require 540 mg/day; children between 1 and 10 years of age, 800 mg/day; adolescents (11 to 18 years), 1200 mg/day; and adults (over 18 years), 800 mg/day (35). More recently, several investigators have shown that whereas these values will allow for certain physiologic needs, they are well below the amount of calcium needed to maintain positive bone balance. Heaney and coworkers (36) found that to be in calcium balance, premenopausal women needed 1000 mg/day; women in the perimenopause, 1200 mg/day, and postmenopausal women, 1400 mg/day. This greater requirement for postmenopausal women is due to a combination of less efficient calcium absorption from the gut and poorer calcium reabsorption by the kidneys. Treatment of postmenopausal women with estrogen results in a better absorptive/reabsorption mechanism, with a resultant decrease in the daily requirement to 1200 mg/day. Spencer and coworkers (37) demonstrated a similar result in men. On a calcium intake of 800 mg/day, 41% of the subjects tested were in negative balance; the incidence decreased to 13% on calcium intakes of 1200 mg/day, and 0% at 1400 mg/day. Based on the present RDA for calcium, the premenopausal requirements for this essential mineral are 25% higher than the RDA, and 75% higher for postmenopausal women. The deficiency of calcium in real terms among the majority of Caucasian postmenopausal women is actually greater: Avioli (38) and others (39,40) have shown that the average intake of calcium by women between the ages of 40 and 65 varies between 450 and 600 mg/day. Thus, the average daily calcium intake should be increased by 100%!

Calcium is absorbed primarily in the small intestine in a gradient that is maximal in the duodenum and proximal jejunum. Absorption of calcium is completed within 4 hours of its intake and is due to a combination of three processes: (1) passive diffusion, (2) binding by transfer to a protein carrier, and (3) active transport. With a low calcium intake, the absorption of calcium is said to become more efficient. This process is referred to as adaptation and is exhibited to a greater extent in younger than in older persons. Whereas 75% of ingested calcium may be absorbed by children during periods of rapid skeletal growth and remodeling, the value decreases to 30 to 50% in adults (41). Intestinal calcium absorption decreases even more in elderly women (over the age of 70), and especially in women with osteoporosis (42).

Despite contrary opinions, calcium is absorbed as efficiently from calcium supplements as it is from food sources known to be rich in calcium, such as dairy products. In carefully performed calcium balance studies, Spencer and coworkers (37) were able to establish that it was the amount of available calcium and not the source (milk versus calcium gluconate) that determined whether an individual would achieve calcium balance. The most important point is that the calcium requirement is needed consistently on a daily basis; as with exercise, individuals need to be given the option of meeting this essential daily need by whatever means is convenient, acceptable, and affordable. In an ongoing study at The Center for Climacteric Studies (involving 92 women in the 2 year exercise program to prevent osteoporosis), it was found that initially only 41% of the women met the RDA of calcium and 12%, the desired 1400 mg of calcium required per day. With successive interviews, significant increases in calcium intake were observed. By the fifth interview, at 12 months, 93% of women met the RDA and 82%, the 1400 mg requirement. The desired calcium intake of 1400 mg was met from food sources in 8% of the women. Reasons given for not increasing calcium-rich foods include concern for weight gain, lactose intolerance, dislike of certain dairy products, and constipation.

Much is written about the preferred or best type of calcium supplement; basic to the issue, however, is compliance. The fewer tablets (and the least expensive), the more likely it will be that an individual will take the supplement. In this context, two essential points need emphasis:

1. It is only elemental calcium that is available for absorption; calcium carbonate contains 40% of calcium in this form, calcium lactate 13%, and calcium gluconate 9%. Studies by Spencer and coworkers (37) showed that the availability of calcium from these sources does not differ significantly. Fewer calcium carbonate tablets will be needed to deliver a given amount of calcium; compliance should, therefore, be enhanced.

2. The timing of calcium supplementation can theoretically maximize its absorption. The division of calcium intake into multiple feedings is less likely to saturate the intestinal absorptive mechanism (41); calcium also has a diurnal metabolism—it is stored in bone during the day and released during the night (43), when it is needed to provide for the systemic needs of the individual at a time when there is no dietary source. The required amount is taken from the skeleton's soluble calcium pool; by supplementing at night, the drainage from this source of stored calcium may be inhibited or substantially reduced.

Factors Affecting Calcium Metabolism

Bone Robbers. The bioavailability of calcium may be influenced by a number of other nutrients and foods. Dietary fiber binds calcium and prevents its absorption. The addition of cellulose (44) and fruits and vegetables (45) high in fiber creates a negative calcium balance by decreasing absorption of dietary calcium. It is probably the uronic acid residues in hemicellulose that account for the complexing of calcium by dietary fiber. Phytic acid, found in bran and the seed coat of beans and grains, can also reduce calcium absorption; the same is true for oxalic acid, found in vegetables such as spinach. Since dietary oxalate in plant food is already precomplexed with calcium, it will have less of an inhibiting effect on the absorption of other dietary calcium than fiber and phytates. Recent research in rats and in humans has suggested that the colon might play an important role in the conservation of dietary calcium. Since the dietary inhibitors of calcium absorption—phytates, oxalate, and fiber—are metabolized by colonic bacteria, it is possible that the calcium found in the small intestine might be released in the colon and made available for absorption. This has been found to be true for individuals who have required small bowel resections.

Lactase Deficiency. Lactase deficiency may lead to calcium deprivation because of the long-term avoidance of dairy products, such as milk. In one of the best-controlled studies, Newcomer and coworkers (46) found that 27% of women with postmenopausal osteoporosis were lactase deficient, versus 3% of normal women. Although none of the lactase deficient women were overtly aware of milk intolerance, the intake of both lactose (6.5 g/day, versus 17.0 g/day in controls) and calcium (530 mg/day versus 810 mg/day in controls) was significantly lower. Lactase-deficient individuals not only have a decreased calcium intake, but the associated low lactose intake decreases the absorption of calcium from the gut. Lactose deficiency, per se, inhibits calcium absorption (47); conversely, the administration of lactose enhances calcium absorption in normal and even in lactase-deficient subjects (48). A convenient and palatable way of overcoming the problem of lactase deficiency is to advise affected individuals to eat yogurt. Yogurt is manufactured by incubating specialized bacterial organisms with concentrated milk solids. During the process of fermentation, the bacteria produce the lactase enzyme; this allows lactose to be absorbed and with it, calcium. A group of volunteers with a history of lactase deficiency was shown to absorb 50% of the lactose in milk, versus 85% of the lactose in yogurt (49). This improved absorption was also associated with a decrease in abdominal pain and diarrhea.

Dietary Protein and Calcium Balance. Excess amounts of protein have been shown to increase the urinary excretion of calcium. Human volunteers given as much as 1600 mg of calcium per day experienced a negative calcium balance of 140 mg/day on a dietary protein intake of 225g. This negative balance persisted for 48 days without a compensatory increase in the intestinal absorption of calcium or a reduction in the urinary excretion of calcium. If maintained for 1 year, this could lead to a loss of 4% of the total skeletal calcium.

The RDA of protein for adult men is 56 g/day, but the average man consumes more than 100 g, while athletes in training often have intakes in excess of 500g. In premenopausal women there is a significant inverse relationship between nitrogen intake and calcium balance. A 50% increase in protein is associated with a net calcium loss of 32 mg/day (50). Administration of protein to normal subjects increases the urinary calcium excretion and may result in a negative calcium balance (36); the mechanism for this calcium loss may be the sulphur amino acid content of the proteins, which causes a decrease in the renal tubular reabsorption of calcium (51). This effect is not induced by meats, presumably because of the high phosphorus content. Phosphorus decreases urinary calcium excretion (52). Despite this latter observation, it is pertinent to note that lactoovovegetarians have a slow cortical bone loss (53), whereas omnivores, such as Eskimos, are rapid cortical bone losers (54).

Sodium

An excess of dietary sodium in rats is associated with increased PTH secretion and loss of bone (55); a similar feature is noted in humans given more than 2000 mg of sodium (1 teaspoonful) per day (56). In addition, there is a rise in the fasting urinary excretion of sodium as well as calcium after the menopause (57). It is not known whether any of these effects are significant or sufficiently long-lasting to have a real effect on the development of osteopenia. It is conceivable that an excess of dietary sodium could play a secondary role in augmenting bone loss.

Phosphate

A high phosphate intake in rats is associated with secondary hyperparathyroidism and cortical bone loss (58). The same result has been noted in cats and dogs given meat but not the bones usually found in the diet of carnivores.

Although phosphate administration causes an increase in PTH, its effect is not sustained (59). Further, variations in the amount of phosphate ingested and alterations of the phosphate ratio (over and above the ideal calcium/phosphorus ratio of 1/2) in humans does not have an adverse effect on calcium balance (36,60). Despite the fact that the western diet is said to be excessively high in phosphate and phosphate additives, the calcium/phosphorus ratio is actually higher (61) in western societies (0.63) than in countries elsewhere, for example, Colombia, Ecuador, and Jamaica, where the ratio is 0.40 (62). This may be due to the calcium/phosphorus ratio of 1/2.8 found in dairy products—the main dietary source of calcium in western diets.

In a 4 year longitudinal study, Vose, and coworkers (63) reported that osteoporotics given 1 g/day of elemental phosphate had a 0.9% gain in bone compared with a 4.5% loss in controls. There are no studies that relate low bone mass or fractures to the intake of phosphate.

Lifestyle and Calcium Retention

A high caffeine intake—in excess of five cups of coffee per day—increases urinary calcium by an unidentified mechanism (50). Smoking is also associated with a lower bone mass but it is not known whether this is because smokers weigh less, experience an earlier menopause, or suffer from chronic pulmonary disease and systemic acidosis (64). Bone loss resulting from alcohol excess (65) may be due to a combination of factors: poor nutrition, including an inadequate intake of calcium and vitamin D, gastrointestinal and pancreatic malfunction, a deficiency of activated vitamin D as a result of liver impairment, and a defect in the hydroxylation of the provitamin to its partially activated form have all been incriminated. Alcohol also inhibits the absorption of calcium from the gut (66).

Inactivity and immobilization result in a significant increase in both urinary and fecal calcium excretion (67); this is compounded by a decrease in calcium absorption associated with immobilization (68). Conversely, exercise decreases the hypercalciuria induced by immobilization and results in a reversal of the negative calcium balance (69).

Some medications can also interfere with calcium metabolism. Aluminum-containing antacids enhance urinary calcium and fecal calcium excretion. This is brought about by phosphorus depletion and secondary calcium loss. The phosphorus deficiency is caused by the formation of complexes between the aluminum and dietary phosphorus in the intestines. This effect is noticeable with relatively small doses (90 ml/day) of these antacids (70). Other medications that may lead to hypercalciuria include glucocorticoids, certain diuretics (furosemide), tetracycline, and the long-term use of the antituberculosis drug isoniazid.

Vitamin D. Elderly patients and women with osteporosis absorb calcium less efficiently. This is thought to be due to a deficiency of the activated form of vitamin D, 1,25 $(OH)_2$ D_3—calcitriol (42), and illustrates the well-known fact that vitamin D is a major factor for the absorption of calcium and for the maintenance of calcium balance.

Because vitamin D is synthesized in the skin in response to solar irradiation, its significance as a nutrient is frequently underestimated. A reduced dietary intake, especially if associated with intestinal malabsorption of fats, could result in the depletion of vitamin D stores in elderly persons not exposed to sunlight.

Subclinical vitamin D depletion may predispose the elderly to hip fractures as a result of accelerated cortical bone loss associated with secondary hyperparathyroidism.

Despite this, excess amounts of vitamin D may be even more harmful and lead to an increase in urinary calcium excretion and a further loss of cortical bone (71). It is currently recommended that dietary and/or supplemental vitamin D should not exceed 1000 IU/day.

Fluoride. The use of fluorides stems from the observation of increased skeletal radiopacity in individuals living in areas with a high fluoride content in the drinking water. A population study in North Dakota showed that the prevalence of osteoporosis was lower in communities with a higher water content of fluoride (72). Similar observations have been made in other areas of the United States and elsewhere. It appears that individuals who live in areas where the water contains four to six parts per million of fluoride, will have increased bone density.

Fluoride affects bone in two ways:

1. The fluoride ion replaces the hydroxyapatite with fluorapatite, producing a mineral of greater crystallinity that is more resistant to resorption.
2. Fluoride stimulates osteoblastic activity. The increased formation of osteoid necessitates mineralization with calcium; if calcium is not provided, the newly formed bone will be indistinguishable from osteomalasic bone, and could result in a high incidence of fractures, especially in the cortical bone, for example, the femur (33).

If fluoride is given in high doses (50 to 60 mg of sodium fluoride per day), together with calcium in appropriate doses, new bone formation will occur and vertebral fractures will be prevented. A decrease in the fracture rate will be noted only after 1 or 2 years' treatment (74), but symptomatic improvement with decreased pain and increased movement has been noted within 12 weeks (75). Unfortunately, only about one-third of subjects will respond to this form of treatment; one-third will show no response, while the remainder will experience severe side effects—arthralgias, plantar fasciitis, gastrointestinal upsets, and reactivation of peptic ulcer disease—that will necessitate discontinuance of treatment.

Although prolonged fluoride therapy may result in fluorosis, no cases have been reported to date. To ensure safe and effective supplementation with fluoride, normal kidney function is obligatory; the fluoride should be taken in divided doses with meals and at a time separate from the added calcium. If taken together, the fluoride and calcium will form an insoluble complex that will preclude the absorption of either compound.

The use of fluoride is experimental and has not been approved by the FDA for treatment of osteoporosis. However, when fluoride is combined with appropriate doses of estrogen, calcium, and vitamin D, the incidence of recurrent vertebral fractures has been reduced by 83% in some studies (76).

NUTRITION AND OSTEOPOROSIS PREVENTION: CLINICAL EXPERIENCE

There are no long-term longitudinal studies that have shown a decrease in the incidence of osteoporosis-related fractures due to nutritional intervention. However, many studies strongly suggest that calcium plays a role in the prevention of osteoporosis. Thus, in a recent community study, Matkovic and coworkers (77) compared individuals from a high calcium area in Yugoslavia (Podravina), and a neighboring low calcium district (Istra). The average calcium intakes were 0.48 g/day and 1.01 g/day in the younger population from the low and high calcium areas, respectively, and 0.37 and 0.89 g/day in the older group. The populations were comparable in all other respects. Peak adult cortical bone mass was decreased in the low calcium population by about 5% in women and 10% in men. The low calcium community also had a significantly high incidence of fractures of the femur. This study illustrates the importance of acquiring peak bone mass before the physiologic postmenopausal bone-losing phase.

Riggs and coworkers (76), in a retrospective analysis of patients managed according to different regimens, noted that treatment with 1.5 to 2.5 g of calcium carbonate per day (plus vitamin D in 70% of the patients) led to a vertebral fracture rate one-half that observed in untreated patients. Short-term longitudinal studies (78) have shown that 1.2 g/day of calcium resulted in a lesser decrease in the cortical area of metacarpals than in untreated controls (0.06 mm^2/year versus 0.26 mm^2/year) and no deterioration of the spinal vertebral fracture score. A similar result was supported by Recker and coworkers (79) who gave 1.0 g/day to postmenopausal women for 2 years; once again, the treatment group lost less cortical (measured by metacarpal radiogrammetry) and mixed trabecular/cortical bone from the distal radius (measured by single photon absorptiometry). The calcium balance in the treated group was seven times less negative than in the control group (79). Trials that provided supplemental calcium in 0.5 g/day dosage did not conserve bone mass (80,81) It would seem that a calcium supplement of 1.0 g/day or more is needed for a clinical effect to occur.

Two histomorphometric studies using quantitative microradiography illustrated that patients on calcium supplement (1.5 to 2.5 g/day) exhibited a significant decrease in bone resorbing surfaces 4 months (82), and 2 years after treatment (83). The mechanism of action of calcium supplements is not known. Postulates include a decrease in the sensitivity of bone to PTH and an increase in the bone-conserving hormone calcitonin (84). An interesting recent report (85) has shown that a 1.0 g calcium supplement decreased the hydroxyprotein/creatine ratio in postmenopausal women with osteoporosis from 0.002 to 0.017 ($p < .005$) indicating a significant reduction in bone resorption, and possibly protection of the protein matrix.

The only potential adverse side effect of calcium therapy is renal stones. They rarely develop in women and when they do occur, are found in individuals who lack the enzymes necessary to keep the calcium and urine in solution, and not because of an excessive intake of calcium. In any event, the 24 hour urinary excretion of calcium should be monitored and kept below 300 mg/day; with a high fluid intake, the calcium concentration in urine can be kept at a level incompatible with renal stone formation.

Most of the other nutrients, for example, vitamin D, phosphate, protein, and sodium, probably play a supplementary role in maintaining bone mass, but could have a negative impact on bone homeostasis if present in either very low or very high amounts.

Osteoporosis has been aptly referred to as a "silent epidemic." There are no overt clinical signs of this condition before fracturing actually occurs. It has reached epidemic proportions as a consequence of increasing longevity, compounded by lifestyles that have led to women's reaching their menopause with an inadequate bone mineral reserve.

It is essential to appreciate that osteoporosis is a complex, multifactoral condition. Nevertheless, by educating the public about osteoporosis and applying the basic principles of bone physiology to our everyday activity and needs, much can be done to ensure against later development of this asymptomatic disease. Two goals need to be reached: acquire as much bone as possible before the menopause; modulate the rate of bone loss thereafter.

These goals can be achieved by appropriate and consistent exercise to stimulate new bone; a balanced diet to maximize bone mineralization; and moderation in lifestyle habits, for example, smoking, alcohol, and caffeine excess, to regulate the rate at which bone is lost.

It is not normal for our senior citizens to be transformed by ageing into "little old ladies." If practiced from an early age, good bone hygiene can insure that all women can share in the right to *Stand Tall*.

REFERENCES

1. A. F. Lewis, *Brit. Med. J.*, **283,** 1217 (1981).
2. J. S. Keene and C. A. Anderson, *J.A.M.A.*, **248,** 564 (1982).
3. A. M. Parfitt, in R. Recker, Ed., *Bone Histomorphometry. Techniques and Interpretation*, C.R.C. Press, Boca Raton, 1983, p. 143.
4. P. Tran Van, A. Vignery, and R. Baron, *Cell. Tis. Res.*, **225,** 283 (1982).
5. M. Owen, *Arth. Rheum.*, **23,** 1073 (1980).
6. S. Mohan, T. Linkhart, J. Farley, and D. Baylink, *Calcif. Tis. Int.*, **36,** S139 (1984).
7. J. L. Katz, H. J. Yoon, S. Lipson, et al., *Calcif. Tis., Int.*, **36,** S31 (1984).

8. C. Nagent de Deuxchaisnes, in A. St. J. Dixon, R. G. G. Russel, and T. C. Stump, Eds., *Osteoporosis: A Multidisciplinary Problem*, Academic, London, 1983, p. 291.
9. B. L. Riggs, H. W. Wahner, W. C. Dunn, et al., *J. Clin. Invest.*, **67,** 328 (1981).
10. D. R. Carter, W. C. Hayes, and A. Schurman, *J. Biomech.*, **9,** 211 (1976).
11. D. R. Carter, *Calcif. Tis. Int.*, **36,** S19 (1984).
12. Editorial, *Lancet,* **2,** 1365 (1983).
13. R. Krølner and B. Toft, *Clin. Sci.,* **64,** 537 (1983).
14. F. E. Tilton, J. J. C. Degioanni, and V. S. Schneider, *Aviation, Space and Environ. Med.,* **51,** 1209 (1980).
15. G. D. Whedon, in P. L. White and T. Mondeika, Eds., *Diet and Exercise: Synergism in Health Maintenance*, American Med. Asso., Chicago 1982, p. 99.
16. B. E. Nilsson and N. E. Westlin, *Clin. Orthop.*, **77,** 179 (1971).
17. N. Dalen and K. E. Olsson, *Acta. Orthop. Scan.*, **45,** 170 (1974).
18. B. E. Nilsson, S. M. Anderson, T. Havdrup, and N. E. Westlin, *Am. J. Roentgenol.*, **131,** 539 (1978).
19. J. F. Aloia, S. H. Cohn, J. A. Ostuni, et al., *Ann. Intern. Med.*, **89,** 356 (1978).
20. E. L. Smith, W. Reddan, and P. E. Smith, *Med. Sci. Sports Exerc.*, **13,** 60 (1981).
21. B. Krølner, B. Toft, S. P. Nielsen, and E. Tondenvold, *Clin. Sci.,* **64,** 541 (1983).
22. E. L. Smith, P. E. Smith, C. J. Ensign, and M. M. Shea, *Calcif. Tis. Int.*, **36,** S129 (1984).
23. L. E. Lanyon, *Calcif. Tis. Int.*, **36,** S56 (1984).
23(a). R. A. Yeater and R. B. Martin, Postgrad. Med., **75,** 147 (1984).
24. S. L. Y. Woo, S. C. Kuei, D. Amiel, et al., *J. Bone Joint Surg.,* **63A,** 780 (1980).
25. L. Emiola and J. P. O'Shea, *Nutr. Rep. Int.*, **17,** 669 (1978).
26. A. Kiiskinen, *Growth*, **41**:123 (1977).
27. B. L. Drinkwater, K. Nilson, C. Chestnut, et al., *N. Engl. J. Med.*, **311,** 277 (1984).
28. C. E. Cann, M. C. Martin, H. K. Genant, and R. B. Jaffe, *J.A.M.A.*, **251,** 626 (1984).
29. V. Brewer, B. M. Meyer, M. S. Keele, et al., *Med. Sci.* Sports Exerc., **15,** 445 (1983).
30. N. A. Rigotti, S. R. Nussbaum, D. B. Herzog, and R. M. Neer, *N. Engl. J. Med.*, **311,** 1601 (1984).
31. Z. Davidovitch, J. L. Shanfeld, P. C. Montgomery, et al., *Calcif. Tis. Int.*, **36,** S86 (1984).
32. I. Binderman, Z. Shimshoni, and D. Somjen, *Calcif. Tis. Int.*, **36,** S82 (1984).
33. M. Chvapil, D. Bartos, and F. Bartos, *Gerontologia*, **19,** 263 (1973).
34. J. Inkovaara, R. Keikinheimo, K. Jarvinen, et al., Brit. *Med. J.*, **3,** 73 (1975).
35. L. H. Allen, *Curr. Concepts Gastroenterol.,* March/April, 31 (1983).

36. R. P. Heaney, J. C. Gallagher, C. C. Johnston, et al., *Am. J. Clin. Nutr.*, **36,** 986 (1982).
37. H. Spencer, L. Kramer, M. Lesniak, et al., *Clin. Orthoped. Rel. Res.,* **184,** 270 (1984).
38. L. V. Avioli, *Fed. Proc.*, **40,** 2418 (1981).
39. H. H. Draper and C. A. Scythes, *Fed. Proc.*, **40,** 2434 (1981).
40. A. A. Albanese, E. J. Lorenze, and E. H. Wein, *Am. Fam. Phys.,* **18,** 160 (1978).
41. L. V. Avioli, in P. B. Beeson, W. McDermott, and J. B. Wyngaarden, Eds., *Cecil Textbook of Medicine*, Saunders, Philadelphia, 1979, p. 2225.
42. J. C. Gallagher, L. B. Riggs, J. Eisman, et al., *J. Clin. Invest.*, **64,** 729 (1979).
43. A. M. Parfitt, in H. F. de Luca, H. M. Frost, W. S. S. Jee, C. C. Johnston, and A. M. Parfitt, Eds., *Osteoporosis: Recent Advances in Pathogenesis and Treatment*, University Park Press, Baltimore, 1981, p. 115.
44. J. L. Slavin, and J. A. Marlett, *Am. J. Clin. Nutr.*, **33,** 1932 (1980).
45. J. L. Kelsay, K. M. Behall, and E. J. Prather, *Am. J. Clin. Nutr.*, **32,** 1876 (1979).
46. A. D. Newcomer, S. F. Hodgson, D. B. McGill, and P. J. Thomas, *Ann. Int. Med.*, **89,** 218 (1978).
47. E. Greenwald, J. Samachson, and H. Spencer, *J. Nutr.*, **79,** 531 (1963).
48. L. Kramer, H. Spencer, and C. Norris, *Am. J. Clin. Nutr.*, **37,** 713 (1983).
49. J. C. Kolars, M. D. Levitt, M. Aouji, and D. A. Savaiano, *N. Engl. J. Med.*, **310,** 1 (1984).
50. R. P. Heaney, and R. R. Recker, *J. Lab. Clin. Med.*, **99,** 46 (1982).
51. S. J. Whiting, and H. H. Draper, *J. Nutr.*, **111,** 178 (1981).
52. H. Spencer, L. Kramer, M. DeBartolo, et al., *Am. J. Clin. Nutr.*, **37,** 924 (1983).
53. A. G. Marsh, T. V. Sanchez, O. Mickelsen, and G. Mayor, *J. Am. Diet. Assoc.*, **76,** 148 (1980).
54. R. B. Mazess, and W. Mather, *Am. J. Clin. Nutr.*, **27,** 916 (1974).
55. A. Goulding, *Min. Electro. Metab.*, **4,** 203 (1980).
56. C. R. Kleeman, J. Bohannon, D. Bernstein, et al., *Proc. Soc. Exp. Biol. Med.*, **115,** 29 (1964).
57. A. Goulding, *N.Z. Med. J.*, **93,** 924 (1981).
58. H. H. Draper, and R. R. Bell, *Adv. Nutr. Res.*, **2,** 79 (1979).
59. R. R. Bell, H. H. Draper, D. Y. Tzeng, et al., *J. Nutr.*, **107,** 42 (1977).
60. H. Spencer, L. Kramer, D. Osis, and C. Norris, *J. Nutr.*, **108,** 447 (1978).
61. H. H. Draper, and C. A. Scythes, *Fed. Proc.*, **40,** 2434 (1981).
62. B. E. C. Nordin, M. M. Young, L. Bulusu, and A. Horsman, in U.S. Barzel, Ed., *Osteoporosis*, Grune and Stratton, New York, 1970, p. 47.
63. G. P. Vose, D. K. Keele, A. M. Milner, et al., *J. Gerontol.*, **33,** 204 (1978).
64. H. W. Daniell, *Arch. Int. Med.*, **136,** 298 (1976).
65. P. D. Saville, *J. Bone Joint Surg.*, **47A,** 492 (1965).
66. E. L. Drawitt, *Proc. Soc. Exp. Biol. Med.*, **146,** 406 (1974).
67. C. L. Donaldson, S. B. Hulley, J. M. Vogel, et al., *Metabolism*, **19,** 1071 (1970).

68. M. R. Haussler, and T. A. McCain, *N. Engl. J. Med.*, **297,** 974 (1977).
69. A. M. Parfitt, J. C. Gallagher, R. P. Heaney, et al., *Am. J. Clin. Nutr.*, **36,** 1014 (1982).
70. H. Spencer, L. Kramer, C. Norris, and D. Osis, *Am. J. Clin. Nutr.*, **36,** 32 (1982).
71. B. E. C. Nordin, A. Horsman, R. G. Crilly, et al., *Brit. Med. J.*, **280,** 451 (1980).
72. D. S. Bernstein, N. Sadowsky, D. M. Hegsted, et al., *J.A.M.A.*, **198,** 499 (1966).
73. J. E. Compston, S. Chadha, and A. L. Merrett, *Brit. Med. J.*, **281,** 910 (1980).
74. D. Briancon, and P. J. Meunier, *Orthop. Clin. North Am.*, **12,** 629 (1981).
75. O. Grove, and B. Halver, *Acta Med. Scand.*, **209,** 469 (1981).
76. B. L. Riggs, E. Seeman, S. F. Hodgson, et al., *N. Engl. J. Med.*, **306,** 446 (1982).
77. V. Matkivic, K. Kostial, J. Simonovic, et al., *Am. J. Clin. Nutr.*, **32,** 540 (1979).
78. B. E. C. Nordin, A. Horsman, R. G. Crilly, et al., *Brit. Med. J.*, **1,** 451 (1980).
79. R. R. Recker, P. D. Saville, and R. P. Heaney, *Ann. Intern. Med.*, **87,** 649 (1977).
80. C. Christensen, M. S. Christensen, and I. Transbol, *Lancet*, **1,** 459 (1981).
81. C. H. Chestnut, D. J. Baylink, H. E. Gruber, et al., in N. F. deLuca, H. M. Frost, W. S. S. Jee, C. C. Johnston, and A. M. Parfitt, Eds., *Osteoporosis: Recent Advances in Pathogenesis and Treatment*, University Park Press, Baltimore, 1981, p. 411.
82. G. L. Riggs, J. Jowsey, P. J. Kelly, et al., *J. Clin. Endocrinol. Metab.*, **42,** 1139 (1976).
83. R. G. Van Kesteren, S. A. Duursma, W. J. Visser, et al., *Metab. Bone Dis. and Rel. Res.*, **4,** 31 (1982).
84. L. A. Austin, H. Heath, and V. L. W. Go, *J. Clin Invest.*, **64,** 1721 (1979).
85. M. Horwitz, A. G. Need, J. C. Philcox, and B. C. E. Nordin, *Am. J. Clin. Nutr.*, **39,** 857 (1984).

Index